Point-of-Care Testing

Guest Editor

KENT LEWANDROWSKI, MD

CLINICS IN LABORATORY MEDICINE

www.labmed.theclinics.com

Consulting Editor
ALAN WELLS, MD, DMSc

September 2009 • Volume 29 • Number 3

SAUNDERS an imprint of ELSEVIER, Inc.

W.B. SAUNDERS COMPANY
A Division of Elsevier Inc.

1600 John F. Kennedy Boulevard • Suite 1800 • Philadelphia, Pennsylvania 19103-2899

http://www.theclinics.com

CLINICS IN LABORATORY MEDICINE Volume 29, Number 3

September 2009 ISSN 0272-2712, ISBN-13: 978-1-4377-1233-9, ISBN-10: 1-4377-1233-9

Editor: Katie Hartner
Developmental Editor: Donald Mumford

Reprints. For copies of 100 or more, of articles in this publication, please contact the Commercial Reprints Department, Elsevier Inc., 360 Park Avenue South, New York, New York 10010-1710. Tel. (212) 633-3813, Fax: (212) 462-1935, E-mail: reprints@elsevier.com.

Clinics in Laboratory Medicine (ISSN 0272-2712) is published quarterly by Elsevier Inc., 360 Park Avenue South, New York, NY 10010-1710. Months of issue are March, June, September, and December. Business and Editorial offices: 1600 John F. Kennedy Blvd., Suite 1800, Philadelphia, PA 19103-2899. Periodicals postage paid at NewYork, NY and additional mailing offices. Subscription prices are $204.00 per year (US individuals), $321.00 per year (US institutions), $106.00 (US students), $234.00 per year (Canadian individuals), $405.00 per year (foreign institutions), $145.00 (foreign students). Foreign air speed delivery is included in all *Clinics* subscription prices. All prices are subject to change without notice. POSTMASTER: Send address changes to *Clinics in Laboratory Medicine*, Elsevier Health Sciences Division, Subscription Customer Service, 3251 Riverport Lane, Maryland Heights, MO 63043. **Customer Service: 1-800-654-2452 (US). From outside of the US and Canada, call 1-314-447-8871. Fax: 1-314-447-8029. E-mail: journalscustomerservice-usa@elsevier.com (for print support) or journalsonlinesupport-usa@elsevier.com (for online support).**

Clinics in Laboratory Medicine is covered in *EMBASE/Exerpta Medica, MEDLINE/PubMed (Index Medicus), Cinahl, Current Contents/Clinical Medicine, BIOSIS* and *ISI/BIOMED.*

Printed and bound by CPI Group (UK) Ltd, Croydon, CR0 4YY

Transferred to Digital Print 2011

Contributors

GUEST EDITOR

KENT LEWANDROWSKI, MD
Associate Chief of Pathology, Director of Clinical Services (Anatomic and Clinical), Massachusetts General Hospital, Boston, Massachusetts; Associate Professor, Harvard Medical School, Boston, Massachusetts

AUTHORS

DAVID ALTER, MD
Department of Pathology and Laboratory Medicine, Spectrum Health, Grand Rapids, Michigan

T. KEITH BROCK, BS
Department of Pathology and Laboratory Medicine, UC Davis-LLNL Point-of-Care Technologies Center [NIBIB, NIH], Point-of-Care Testing Center for Teaching and Research (POCT•CTR), School of Medicine, University of California, Davis, California

SHELDON CAMPBELL, MD, PhD
Associate Professor, Department of Laboratory Medicine, Yale University School of Medicine, New Haven, Connecticut

GREG DEINES, DO
Center for Diabetes and Endocrinology, Michigan Medical, P.C., Grand Rapids, Michigan

SHARON S. EHRMEYER, PhD, MT(ASCP)
Professor, Director, Clinical Laboratory Science/Medical Technology Program, Department of Pathology and Laboratory Medicine, University of Wisconsin School of Medicine and Public Health, Madison, Wisconsin

YURI FEDORIW, MD
Assistant Professor, Department of Pathology and Laboratory Medicine, Division of Hematopathology, University of North Carolina, School of Medicine Campus, Chapel Hill, North Carolina

ISABEL GAUSS, MT(ASCP)
Department of Clinical Pathology, William Beaumont Hospital, Royal Oak, Michigan; Beaumont Reference Laboratory, William Beaumont Hospital, Royal Oak, Michigan; Department of Pathology, Wayne State University, Detroit, Michigan

NICOLE L. GENTILE, BS
Department of Pathology and Laboratory Medicine, UC Davis-LLNL Point-of-Care Technologies Center [NIBIB, NIH], Point-of-Care Testing Center for Teaching and Research (POCT•CTR), School of Medicine, University of California, Davis, California

KIM GREGORY, MT(ASCP), NCA, CLS
Department of Pathology, Massachusetts General Hospital, Boston, Massachusetts

KRISTIN N. HALE, BS, BA
Department of Pathology and Laboratory Medicine, UC Davis-LLNL Point-of-Care
Technologies Center [NIBIB, NIH], Point-of-Care Testing Center for Teaching and
Research (POCT•CTR), School of Medicine, University of California, Davis, California

CAROL A. HOLLAND, PhD
Beckman Coulter, Inc., High Sensitivity Testing Group, Brea, California

FREDERICK L. KIECHLE, MD, PhD
Department of Clinical Pathology, William Beaumont Hospital, Royal Oak, Michigan;
Beaumont Reference Laboratory, William Beaumont Hospital, Royal Oak, Michigan;
Department of Pathology, Wayne State University, Detroit, Michigan

JI YEON KIM, MD, MPH
Department of Pathology, Massachusetts General Hospital and Harvard Medical School,
Pathology Service, Massachusetts General Hospital, Boston, Massachusetts

TYLER K. KITANO, BS
Department of Pathology and Laboratory Medicine, UC Davis-LLNL Point-of-Care
Technologies Center [NIBIB, NIH], Point-of-Care Testing Center for Teaching and
Research (POCT•CTR), School of Medicine, University of California, Davis, California

GERALD J. KOST, MD, PhD, MS, FACB
Department of Pathology and Laboratory Medicine, UC Davis-LLNL Point-of-Care
Technologies Center [NIBIB, NIH], Point-of-Care Testing Center for Teaching and
Research (POCT•CTR), School of Medicine, University of California, Davis, California

RONALD H. LAESSIG, PhD
Emeritus Professor, Population Health Sciences, Emeritus Director, Wisconsin State
Laboratory of Hygiene, University of Wisconsin School of Medicine and Public Health,
Madison, Wisconsin

ELIZABETH LEE-LEWANDROWSKI, PhD, MPH
Director, Research Core Laboratory, Massachusetts General Hospital, Boston,
Massachusetts; Assistant Professor, Harvard Medical School, Boston, Massachusetts

KENT LEWANDROWSKI, MD
Associate Chief of Pathology, Director Clinical Services (Anatomic and Clinical pathology)
Massachusetts General Hospital, Associate Professor, Harvard Medical School, Boston,
Massachusetts

RICHARD F. LOUIE, PhD
Department of Pathology and Laboratory Medicine, UC Davis-LLNL Point-of-Care
Technologies Center [NIBIB, NIH], Point-of-Care Testing Center for Teaching and
Research (POCT•CTR), School of Medicine, University of California, Davis, California

RICHARD A. McPHERSON, MD
Professor of Pathology, Chair of the Division of Clinical Pathology, Virginia
Commonwealth University, Richmond, Virginia

STACY E.F. MELANSON, MD, PhD
Associate Medical Director Clinical Chemistry, Division of Clinical Laboratories,
Department of Pathology, Brigham and Women's Hospital, Boston, Massachusetts
and Assistant Professor; Harvard Medical School

KIMBERLY W. SANFORD, MD
Assistant Professor of Pathology, Associate Director of Transfusion Medicine, Virginia
Commonwealth University, Richmond, Virginia

NAM K. TRAN, PhD
Department of Pathology and Laboratory Medicine, UC Davis-LLNL Point-of-Care
Technologies Center [NIBIB, NIH], Point-of-Care Testing Center for Teaching and
Research (POCT•CTR), School of Medicine, University of California, Davis, California

ELIZABETH M. VAN COTT, MD
Associate Professor, Harvard Medical School Director, Coagulation Laboratory Medical
Director, Core Laboratory Massachusetts General Hospital, Boston, Massachusetts

Contents

> Point-of-care testing is a rapidly growing area in laboratory medicine. Technologies related to point-of-care testing have unique analytical features and are used in a number of clinical applications. These attributes combined with complex regulatory requirements have made point-of-care testing a true specialty within pathology. Manufacturers continue to develop new point-of-care tests and have consolidated multiple assays to single small handheld or bench-top devices. Enterprise hospital-wide data management systems are available to facilitate improved regulatory compliance and transmit test results into the electronic medical record. Some studies have shown that point-of-care testing can improve clinical outcomes or increase the efficiency of hospital operations. In spite of these developments, many challenges remain. In some cases, the quality of point-of-care tests performed by nonlaboratory personnel does not match that of testing performed in the central laboratory. Data management connectivity remains a significant problem, especially for manually performed tests. Managing a point-of-care program to maintain regulatory compliance is also problematic. For these reasons, the future of point-of-care testing is not entirely clear. The most likely scenario will be a slow but progressive growth of point-of-care testing in the hospital, in the outpatient clinic, and in the home.

> The approach to managing a point-of-care testing (POCT) program has evolved over recent years. Although many of the essential features of early POCT management programs remain intact, contemporary challenges including expansion of the test menu, changing regulatory requirements, and the development of more sophisticated data management connectivity require ongoing adaptation of POCT management programs. Despite improvements in test quality and regulatory compliance, significant challenges for the management of POCT will continue for the foreseeable future.

> Managing patient test data and documenting regulatory compliance for tests performed at the point of care have traditionally been significant problems. In many situations, manual record-keeping has proven entirely

inadequate for maintaining the integrity of the patient medical record or for providing an audit trail for quality assurance activities. Starting in the 1990s, a number of companies began to develop and market point-of-care data management systems. Over time, these data management systems have become increasingly sophisticated. It is now possible to interface multiple point-of-care devices from different manufacturers to a central data manager that is bidirectionally interfaced to the laboratory and hospital information systems. Despite these advances, many challenges remain. True real-time point-of-care "connectivity" across an entire institution has yet to be achieved, and there is still no satisfactory solution for manually performed visually read tests, some of which are commonly performed at the point of care. In the future, wireless point-of-care connectivity solutions hold great promise, but these technologies are yet to be fully developed.

All clinical laboratory testing in the United States is regulated by the Clinical Laboratory Improvement Amendments of 1988 (CLIA'88 or CLIA) and overseen by the Centers for Medicare and Medicaid Services. CLIA profoundly changed the prevailing United States regulatory philosophy by imposing uniform requirements for all clinical laboratory testing regardless of where tests are performed. In the hospital, regulatory compliance is usually ensured by regular inspections of the laboratory by either the Joint Commission or by the College of American Pathologists. These organizations may include requirements beyond the minimum standard mandated by CLIA. This article reviews the status of regulatory compliance of point-of-care testing from a perspective of the current regulations in effect in the United Sates in 2009.

Point-of-care testing (POCT) is usually more expensive on a unit-cost basis than testing performed in a central laboratory. It is difficult to manage POCT and to maintain regulatory compliance, especially in large institutions. However, some POCT technologies have improved patient outcomes (patient self-glucose monitoring in the home, tight glycemic control in intensive care settings) or hospital or emergency department operations (whole-blood cardiac-marker testing and D-dimer testing in emergency departments). In some cases, these outcomes result simply from making a new test available, rather than performing the test at the point of care. In most cases, the rapid turnaround time provided by POCT is the main factor that is ultimately responsible for the improvement in outcomes.

Virological, epidemiologic, and operational barriers have slowed the progress toward effective management and eradication of HIV infection, despite significant advances in diagnosis since the early 1980s. Because early diagnosis profoundly affects the health care and survival of infected/high-risk individuals, and because the time required for conventional testing remains a barrier in many settings, rapid HIV testing has been developed for use both in the clinical laboratory and at the point of care. Recent studies have identified applications, advantages, and limitations of these assays, which may influence the development of new and more effective public health testing and screening protocols. In the United States, the Food and Drug Administration has approved the use of six rapid HIV tests. This review summarizes these modern rapid point-of-care HIV tests and their role in preventing the spread of HIV and in detecting, managing, and treating patients affected by the HIV pandemic.

Sensitive and specific assays are available to detect drugs of abuse at the point of care. This article describes the characteristics of point-of-care devices for drug-of-abuse testing with a focus on clinical utility and patient care. This article is not a comprehensive review of all available point-of-care devices. Instead, it discusses general principles of point-of-care testing for drugs of abuse.

Until recently, inpatient glycemic management focused solely on the diabetic patient with few reported studies that discussed hyperglycemic management of the nondiabetic patient. For the last 35 years, the prevailing notion was that hyperglycemia in the acutely ill nondiabetic inpatient was a consequence of illnesses as well as a marker of its severity. It was also thought to be an adaptive response to injury necessary for survival and not necessarily a prognostic indicator of morbidity or mortality. In this article, we discuss the current school of thought regarding prognostic implications of nondiabetic inpatient hyperglycemia, its management (tight glycemic control), and the relationship of point-of-care testing to tight glycemic control.

Colorectal cancer (CRC) is the third most common cancer in the United States. A reduction in cumulative mortality occurs when patients are routinely screened by fecal occult blood tests (FOBT) and early lesions are removed. These point-of-care tests detect minute amounts of blood released from precancerous and cancerous colon lesions. Positive test results should be followed up with complete diagnostic testing to treat precancerous lesions and diagnose patients at earlier stages of cancer, thereby increasing overall survival. More complex assays are designed to detect genetic changes in cells released from malignant and even pre-malignant lesions. This article provides information on the screening and diagnostic tests available for CRC detection as well as the advantages and disadvantages of each.

Point-of-care (POC) assays are available for a variety of coagulation tests. These assays are generally simple to perform and have a more rapid turn-around time than their central-laboratory counterparts. This article discusses the current status of coagulation POC methodologies, focusing on the potential clinical uses and the limitations of platelet function testing, prothrombin time/international normalized ratio, D-dimer, and activated clotting time (ACT). Additional studies are eagerly awaited regarding potential future uses of POC coagulation testing, including the role of platelet function testing and ACT heparin management systems.

Turnaround time for molecular diagnostic tests is critical in detecting infectious agents, in determining a patient's ability to metabolize a drug or drug class, and in detecting minimal residual disease. These applications would benefit from the development of a point-of-care device for nucleic acid extraction, amplification, and detection. The ideal device would have a low cost per test, use a disposable unit use device for all steps in the assay, be portable, and provide a result that requires no interpretation. The creation of such a device requires miniaturization of current technologies and the use of microfluidics, microarrays, and small-diameter capillary tubes to reduce reagent volumes and simplify heat conduction by convection during nucleic acid amplification. This ideal device may be available in 3 to 5 years and will revolutionize and expand the global availability of molecular diagnostic assays.

Advances in technologies for immunoassay testing have enabled the development of 15-minute whole-blood assays for cardiac markers in the evaluation of patients with acute coronary syndromes (ACS) and congestive heart failure. In many cases, the analytical performance of these assays is equivalent to that of testing in the central laboratory. Rapid whole-blood point-of-care assays for troponin, creatine kinase isoenzyme CK-MB, myoglobin, and B-type natriuretic peptides have facilitated efforts to restructure conventional approaches to ACS and heart failure in the emergency room. Improvements in outcomes, including decreased emergency room and hospital length-of-stay, decreased overall cost, and earlier discharge of low-risk patients, have been documented following implementation of these technologies.

THE CLINICS ARE NOW AVAILABLE ONLINE!

Access your subscription at:
www.theclinics.com

Preface

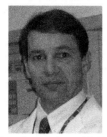

Kent Lewandrowski, MD
Guest Editor

Point-of-care testing (POCT), also called bedside or near-patient testing, is an emerging specialty in laboratory medicine. Attracting considerable interest in the medical literature, POCT is one of the fastest growing areas in laboratory medicine. In this issue, we present a number of articles on the current state of POCT, circa 2009. It has been 8 years since publication of the first issue of *Clinics in Laboratory Medicine: Point-of-Care Testing*. Over this interval, a number of developments have occurred in the applications and practice of POCT. Major trends in the evolution of POCT include:

Expansion of the test menu
Development of more consolidated platforms capable of performing a menu of tests
Emergence of improved analytical technologies that, in some cases, match the performance of central laboratory instruments
Appearance of improved data management systems, including vendor-neutral enterprise connectivity solutions
Progress in making devices easier to use
Advances in enabling patient self-testing in the home
Published demonstrations of improved outcomes (especially those related to operational efficiency) with some types of POCT

As described in the previous issue, the history of POCT has been problematic. In the early 1990s, bedside testing began to make significant inroads in hospitals. Handheld glucose meters originally designed for home patient self-monitoring began to appear in hospital inpatient units for the routine management of diabetic patients during their hospital stay. These devices enabled clinicians to obtain glucose values using a finger-stick capillary blood sample and to make immediate adjustments to insulin dosing without delaying clinical decisions while waiting for test results to return from the clinical laboratory. This capability afforded a level of convenience and timeliness that could not be matched by the central laboratory. Other forms of POCT at the time included fecal occult blood testing, dipstick urinalysis, and urine pregnancy testing. Meanwhile, sundry bedside devices, such as refractometers and urimeters, came into use. At this time, POCT was largely unregulated and few hospitals had an organized structure in place to ensure quality testing. Predictably a number of

Clin Lab Med 29 (2009) xiii–xv
doi:10.1016/j.cll.2009.07.015
0272-2712/09/$ – see front matter © 2009 Elsevier Inc. All rights reserved.

problems began to occur, including those related to quality control, analytical errors, performance of testing by untrained personnel, and lack of proper documentation of patient test results. As a result, hospital and laboratory accreditation agencies began placing increased scrutiny on POCT with more vigorous enforcement of regulatory guidelines mandated by the federal Clinical Laboratory Improvement Amendment (CLIA-88). As POCT became more widespread, it became clear that these technologies were rapidly becoming unmanageable. A number of hospitals experienced embarrassing debacles arising from POCT during routine inspections to renew their laboratory accreditation status. The solution to this problem was to implement formal POCT management teams typically composed of representatives from the laboratory, nursing, and clinical staffs, and from hospital administration.

Initially, laboratory professionals did not embrace POCT. Some of this resistance arose from a genuine concern about the quality of the test results, but a significant part of the issue was concern that POCT would siphon testing out of the clinical laboratory. In the worst-case fear, POCT devices would eventually take over all routine turnaround time–dependant tests and the remainder of the test menu would be sent out to a reference laboratory. This scenario, of course, never materialized. The conventional wisdom a decade ago was that POCT was too expensive, that test results were unreliable, and that POCT was impossible to manage across a hospital campus. Some aspects of these perceptions were true.

From a technology perspective, efforts to improve quality and automate regulatory compliance were spearheaded by the manufacturers of bedside glucose-testing devices, which were, and continue to be, the dominant POCT technology. Several generations of improved devices and software solutions for data management were introduced to solve many of the problems associated with analytical errors and management of testing data. Other vendors developed vendor-neutral open-architecture enterprise-level POCT data management solutions capable of interfacing to multiple devices from different manufacturers. Collectively, these data management solutions significantly improved our ability to manage POCT across the hospital campus and at remote affiliated sites. However, POCT data management and connectivity remains a work in progress particularly for visually read manually performed POCT tests, for which there is currently no satisfactory solution.

Manufacturers have continued to develop new devices and tests designed for applications at the point of care. The fundamental concept underlying POCT is turnaround time. POCT offers the ability to obtain test results at the moment medical decisions must be made. To the extent that timely laboratory test results are essential to many clinical decisions, rapid turnaround time has great conceptual appeal. Yet few published studies have documented improved medical outcomes following implementation of POCT. However, the literature abounds with documentation of the ability of POCT to improve efficiency and to benefit hospital operations. Ironically, although POCT was originally conceived as a mechanism to improve medical outcomes, most of the documented benefits relate to promoting the efficiency of clinical care.

As technologies have improved and more evidence has accumulated that POCT can benefit clinical operations, acceptance of POCT by the laboratory profession has increased. Most laboratory professionals now view POCT as one tool in their arsenal to provide laboratory services to their health care system. The other tools include sending specimens out to reference laboratories and performing testing in a centralized clinical laboratory. Each of these options is appropriate in certain situations but not in others. For example, bedside capillary glucose testing is used almost universally in American hospitals for routine management of diabetic inpatients. Few laboratory professionals would consider eliminating this technology because without it clinical care would be impaired and the laboratory would be regularly flooded with stat glucose requests several times a day. On the other hand, routine testing for thyroid disease at the point of care would be expensive and inappropriate. This testing is most logically performed in a central laboratory. Finally, esoteric low-volume tests not highly dependent on turnaround time (eg, fractionated urine catecholamines) are most efficiently performed in a reference laboratory. The current typical laboratory test menu is large and expanding rapidly. It is the task of laboratory professionals to determine the most clinically and financially appropriate solutions to provide comprehensive laboratory services. POCT represents one possible solution.

The future of POCT is difficult to predict but will be influenced by many of the factors affecting laboratory medicine more generally, such as regulatory issues, pressure for cost containment, evolving clinical needs, improvements in technology, and shortages of trained laboratory technologists. As the population of the United States continues to grow and to age, demographics will likely create more demand for laboratory services. The most likely future scenario will be steady and continued growth of POCT as new technologies are developed and as more tests become available in point-of-care formats. The ability of POCT to improve workflow on clinical services will likely be a major factor as pressure for cost containment will promote health care models that emphasize smooth, efficient operations.

I wish to thank the various authors who have contributed articles to this issue. Without their contributions and expertise, this issue would not have been possible. I also want to thank the publisher, Elsevier, for sponsoring the *Clinics in Laboratory Medicine* series and their commitment to continuing medical education.

Finally, a dedication: to Nicole Lewandrowski, for giving me encouragement when I need it most.

Kent Lewandrowski, MD
Massachusetts General Hospital
Harvard Medical School
55 Fruit Street, Gray 5 Chemistry
Boston, MA 02114, USA

E-mail address:
klewandrowski@partners.org (K. Lewandrowski)

Point-of-Care Testing: An Overview and a Look to the Future (Circa 2009, United States)

Kent Lewandrowski, MD

KEYWORDS

- Point-of-care testing • Near patient testing • History
- Regulatory compliance • Quality control

Point-of-care testing (POCT, also called bedside or near-patient testing) is an emerging specialty in laboratory medicine and has attracted considerable interest in the medical literature. Compared with testing performed in the clinical laboratory, POCT is one of the most rapidly growing areas in laboratory medicine. At the same time, POCT remains controversial, in part because these technologies challenge the conventional approach to laboratory testing. Many of the current uses of POCT are discussed elsewhere in this issue or in the first issue of *Point-of-Care Testing* in 2001.[1] In this issue, authors describe their experiences with POCT, including those related to medical, operational, and regulatory issues. Individual authors may express opinions that differ from those in other articles, which should be expected given their diverse backgrounds and perspectives. This article provides an overview of general concepts relating to POCT and serves as background for the articles that follow.

The first issue of *Clinics In Laboratory Medicine: Point of Care Testing* was published in 2001.[1] The contents included a general overview of important topics relating to POCT, such as cardiac markers, regulatory compliance, and provider-performed microscopy, and other articles on specific POCT applications (**Box 1**).

Since publication of the first issue, there have been many new developments in the field of POCT. This second issue on POCT was planned as an update to the first issue to highlight important new developments and applications for POCT. Included are

This article has been adapted in part from the introduction to the previous *Clinics In Laboratory Medicine Point-Of-Care Testing* and from: Lee-Lewandrowski E, Lewandrowski K. Point-of-Care Testing. In: McClatchey K, editor. Clinical Laboratory Medicine. 2nd Edition. Baltimore (MD): Williams and Wilkins; 2000.

Department of Pathology, Director Clinical Services (Anatomic and Clinical Pathology), Massachusetts General Hospital, Harvard Medical School, 55 Fruit Street, Gray 5 Chemistry, Boston, MA 02114, USA
E-mail address: klewandrowski@partners.org

Box 1
Article topics from the first issue of Clinics in Laboratory Medicine: Point-of-Care Testing

Regulatory compliance for POCT

Management of a POCT program

Cost issues and impact on hospital operations

Impact on medical outcomes

Bedside glucose testing

Acute care testing: blood gases and electrolytes

Coagulation

Cardiac markers

Toxicology and drugs of abuse

Provider-performed microscopy

Selected topics in POCT

---

updates of previous articles addressing such topics as cardiac markers, drugs-of-abuse testing, and regulatory compliance; selected articles on new applications of existing technologies (tight glycemic control); and, finally, new articles on such topics as molecular diagnostics, rapid HIV testing, POCT in disaster management, and informatics/connectivity. Some articles from the first issue have not been repeated (eg, blood gases and electrolytes, bedside glucose testing) because, in the opinion of the editor, significant new advances have not occurred over the interval between issues. For more information on these topics, the reader is referred to the first issue and to the textbooks listed in the references of this article. Concerning the articles in the second issue of *Point-of-Care Testing*, some selected comments are in order:

POCT for cardiac markers in acute coronary syndromes and heart failure: Significant new developments have occurred in the area of POCT cardiac markers. First, several studies have been published documenting improved outcomes resulting from POCT for cardiac markers, including a decrease in emergency department length of stay, more rapid discharge of low-risk patients, and decreased cost for medical care. Analytical technologies have also improved, particularly for cardiac troponins. Finally, POCT devices for measuring B-type natriuretic peptide have been introduced to aid in the diagnosis and management of acute heart failure.

POCT in coagulation: Major developments in POCT coagulation include improvements to the analytical technologies, more widespread patient self-testing for prothrombin time–international normalized ratio in the home, and the introduction of new technologies to evaluate platelet function.

HIV testing near the patient: Several manufacturers have developed rapid whole-blood (or salivary) tests for HIV. These technologies permit immediate assessment of patients suspected of having HIV infection in the clinic or in the emergency department. To the extent that many patients infected with HIV are unaware of their condition, these rapid tests may facilitate identification of patients with unknown HIV infection, ensuring timely referral to appropriate treatment programs.

Fecal occult blood testing: In recent years, several manufacturers have introduced immunochemical methods for assessment of fecal occult blood in colorectal cancer screening programs. These tests were intended to replace traditional guaiac-based testing in which the rate of false-positive results has proven problematic. Considerable effort is being directed to developing formal screening programs for colorectal cancer and these new tests may play a significant role in these efforts.

Tight glycemic control: Bedside glucose testing is used almost universally for routine management of diabetic patients during their hospital stay. However, it has subsequently been observed that maintaining tight glycemic control in acute care settings may significantly reduce morbidity and mortality even in nondiabetic patients.

Drugs-of-abuse testing at the point-of-care: Drugs-of-abuse testing at the point-of-care has been available for many years. Recent developments, which have included expansion of the test menu to include such drugs as tricyclic antidepressants and acetaminophen, have improved the utility of these devices in the acute toxicology setting. Instruments are also now available to read the test results and transmit the data electronically into the medical record.

POCT and molecular diagnostics: New assays using molecular diagnostic techniques allow for improved diagnosis in a number of genetic disorders, in oncology, and in microbiology. Although these techniques are not currently available in true point-of-care formats, many companies are working on assays that may soon bring molecular diagnostics to the point-of-care. The most promising area is molecular microbiology for viral and bacterial pathogens.

Articles on management, regulatory compliance, informatics, cost, and outcomes: These articles provide current perspectives on important topics in POCT unrelated to specific tests or devices. All of these areas have been evolving over the years and require a fresh perspective.

POCT: A HISTORICAL PERSPECTIVE

POCT has been used in various forms for a number of decades and, indeed, since ancient times when practitioners advocated the tasting of urine samples as a test for diabetes mellitus. For a long time, POCT existed under the radar screen of the laboratory profession and was limited to a few tests, such as dipstick urinalysis, physician-performed microscopy, and fecal occult blood testing. Then in the late 1980s, several companies developed simple handheld glucose meters. These devices were intended for home use to assist patients with diabetes mellitus in self-monitoring their own blood glucose values, replacing the less-accurate urine dipstick tests for detecting glycosuria. Several successive generations of devices were produced with improved accuracy and ease of use. In many respects, capillary blood glucose testing revolutionized diabetic management, permitting patients to achieve better control of their glucose values. Tighter glycemic control is directly linked to improved outcomes, reducing diabetic complications, such as diabetic nephropathy, retinopathy, and cardiovascular disease.

In the early 1990s, handheld glucose meters originally designed for home use began to find their way into hospital settings as an aid to manage diabetic patients during their hospital stay. The ability of clinical staff to adjust insulin dosages by rapidly measuring a patient's glucose value at the bedside using a simple finger-stick capillary blood sample provided a level of convenience and timeliness that the central clinical laboratory could not match. Bedside capillary glucose monitoring rapidly became standard of care in the overwhelming majority of general hospitals.

As bedside glucose testing became more widespread, significant issues arose in short order concerning the reliability of POCT, including issues related to accuracy, operator training, quality control, and the management of testing data in the medical record.[2] Passage and eventual implementation of the 1988 Clinical Laboratory Improvement Amendments (CLIA) resulted in the formulation of regulatory guidelines to ensure the quality of POCT. The federal regulations prompted increased scrutiny of POCT from hospital and laboratory accreditation agencies, such as the Joint Commission and the College of American Pathologists. Physician-office POCT came under the scrutiny of the Commission On Laboratory Accreditation, state departments of public health, and other organizations. It soon became apparent that other types of testing beyond blood glucose monitoring (eg, fecal occult blood testing, dipstick urinalysis, rapid strep A testing) fell under the purview of these new and evolving regulations. Perhaps no other area of clinical pathology has been so significantly affected by issues concerning regulatory compliance as POCT. Although these regulations have done much to improve the quality and oversight of POCT, excessive regulation in some situations has slowed innovation and delayed potential improvements in patient care.[3]

For the clinical pathologist responsible for providing laboratory services, there are three options for performing a test: reference laboratories, hospital laboratories, or testing at the point-of-care.[1] Reference laboratories include national commercial operations, such as Quest Diagnostics and Laboratory Corporation of America. These laboratories boast a large test menu and economies of scale owing to the volume of testing performed. Economies of scale translate into a low unit cost (although charges may be much greater). The major disadvantage of reference laboratories is their remoteness, which results in long turnaround times that may be inappropriate for many types of testing. At the opposite end of the spectrum is POCT. In the case of POCT, the available menu is limited and the economies of scale are minimal because tests are performed one at a time. Consequently, the unit cost of POCT tends to be higher than that of alternatives. However, POCT permits rapid turnaround time for test results, which may improve the efficiency and effectiveness of clinical care. The hospital laboratory presents another option. Some hospital laboratories have grown to impressive size with large menus, automated instrumentation, and significant economies of scale. In this respect, hospital laboratories may resemble regional reference operations. Many hospitals have set up stat laboratories and urgent care facilities with pneumatic tube systems to facilitate rapid transport and short turnaround time. These stat laboratories provide a reasonable alternative to POCT in many applications, and may offer some cost and quality advantages. The needs of each institution for laboratory testing are highly variable, depending on geography, available infrastructure, logistics, the type of medical services, patient acuity, reimbursement, regulatory requirements, and a variety of other factors. The three options for providing laboratory testing (reference laboratories, hospital laboratories, and POCT) compete to serve the needs of the patient and physician. Many solutions are possible, depending on a number of complex and at times contradictory factors. In the final analysis, most hospitals use all three options to a greater or lesser degree. Currently a number of tests are now commonly performed at the point-of-care (**Box 2**).

Enthusiasm concerning the opportunities provided by POCT to achieve rapid turnaround time has resulted in substantial and continued investment in POCT technologies by the diagnostics industry.[1] At the same time, hospitals are learning how to manage POCT performed by nonlaboratory personnel using interdisciplinary teams composed of the laboratory, nursing, and hospital administration. Consequently, opportunities to implement successful POCT programs have been expanding as

---

Box 2
Examples of tests commonly performed at the point-of-care

Bedside glucose testing

Blood gases and electrolytes

Coagulation, including activated clotting time

Cardiac markers

Hemoglobin A1c

Physician-performed microscopy

Fecal occult blood testing

Dipstick urinalysis

Urine pregnancy testing

Intraoperative parathyroid hormone

Infectious disease testing: Rapid strep A, influenza A/B, respiratory syncytial virus, HIV

---

technology has progressively improved. Major trends in the evolution of POCT include the following:

Expanded test menus
Consolidated platforms capable of performing a wide menu of tests
Improved analytic technologies in some cases matching performance of central laboratory instruments
Improved data management systems, including multivendor enterprise connectivity solutions
Improved management of POCT using multidisciplinary teams
Improved device ease-of-use with near error-free operation
Increased patient self-testing in the home
Published evidence demonstrating improved outcomes with some types of POCT

In spite of these advances, POCT continues to present major challenges, however, including those related to cost, medical necessity, analytical quality, performance of tests by nonlaboratory personnel, the impact of POCT on hospital operations, and regulatory concerns.

REGULATORY COMPLIANCE

Compliance with regulatory guidelines concerning POCT has proved challenging in many institutions. Most physicians and nurses have little if any training in quality laboratory practices and may fail to appreciate the importance of quality control and proper documentation. However, institutions must comply with POCT regulations to maintain their accreditation status. Predictably, a number of hospitals have experienced embarrassing debacles during routine inspections to renew their accreditation. The solution to the challenge of regulatory compliance was to establish hospital POCT management teams. These teams are usually led by the clinical laboratory in collaboration with representatives from nursing and the clinical community.[4]

Compliance with requirements for documentation is difficult when using handwritten records. For this reason, a number of vendors have developed computer-based "connectivity" solutions to manage test-related data. Several vendors offer enterprise-level POCT data management systems capable of connecting to numerous devices from different manufacturers. These "connectivity" solutions have made regulatory compliance much more manageable for instrument-read tests. However, off-the-shelf interfaces for some POCT instruments are not always readily available. In other cases, the volume of testing performed on a device is too low to cost-justify a purchase or he creation of an interface. In either event, global connectivity for POCT is not yet a reality and will take years to achieve. The result is that managing regulatory compliance for POCT will remain costly and challenging.

QUALITY CONTROL

Another major development to improve regulatory compliance was alternative quality control. Traditional forms of quality control such as multilevel liquid quality control are, with few exceptions, too cumbersome to be practical for POCT. Initially, some vendors developed what became known as electronic quality control (e-QC). These technologies checked the electronics of the device but not the actual testing reagents. The concept was based on demonstration that the reagents were stable from the time of manufacture to the time of use, assuming proper storage conditions. This approach eliminated the need for frequent liquid quality control and greatly facilitated performance and management of POCT. Further development led to automatic quality control (auto-QC), in which liquid quality control is automatically performed by the instrument without the need for operator intervention. This approach provides the convenience of e-QC with the assurance of verifying reagent integrity afforded by liquid quality control. Finally, for devices that still require regular liquid quality control, some instruments are programmed to lock out the user if quality control has not been performed or other failures are detected, such as use of the device by untrained users or the use of expired reagents. The process of performing and documenting quality control has therefore been greatly simplified. Unfortunately, many POCT tests are manually performed and visually read devices, such as devices for fecal occult blood testing and urine pregnancy testing. These devices usually have built-in positive (and in some cases negative) controls performed automatically with each test. However, documenting quality control and patient test results is challenging. There is currently no satisfactory solution to reliably manage test data for manually performed visually read tests other than to develop reader devices to enable electronic data transmission using direct computer interfaces. In many cases, reader devices are not available such that hand written records still must be used.

CURRENT STATUS OF POCT

Despite regulatory and financial obstacles, over time the use of POCT outside of the main clinical laboratory has become standard of care in some situations (bedside glucose testing, activated clotting time). In other situations, POCT is now a viable alternative to the central laboratory in hospital and outpatient settings. For many tests on the laboratory menu, there is now a choice between the central laboratory and POCT. The decision of which tests to offer in the POCT format depends on a number of factors. The most important of these factors is turnaround time. The need for urgent results may arise for clinical reasons (eg, hematocrit in trauma patients), but more often is due to the impact of turnaround time on workflow and hospital operations. The ability to obtain a test result quickly in the course of clinical care potentially avoids costly delays as patients progress through their hospitalization or outpatient visit.

The menu of tests available at the point-of-care continues to grow rapidly (**Box 3**).

Box 3
Partial list of tests available at the point-of-care

Chemistry

Glucose

Blood gases and electrolytes

Lactate

Cholesterol

Hemoglobin A1c

Microalbumin[a]

Basic metabolic panel[a]

Lipid panel[a]

Liver function panel[a]

Cardiac markers (including natriuretic peptides[a])

Urinalysis

Urea nitrogen

Creatinine

Ionized calcium

Drugs of abuse

Pregnancy testing

Infertility testing

Fetal fibronectin[a]

Hematology

Prothrombin time

Partial thromboplastin time

Activated clotting time

Platelet function[a]

D-dimer[a]

Complete blood count

Microbiology

Physician-performed microscopy

Helicobacter pylori testing

Influenza testing[a]

Respiratory syncytial virus[a]

Sexually transmitted diseases (gonorrhea, chlamydia)

HIV[a]

Other

Fecal occult blood

Gastric occult blood

Immunochemical methods for occult blood[a]

[a] Additions to the menu since the first issue of *Clinics* on this topic

Manufacturers have continued to invest in the development of new and upgraded POCT devices and tests. Examples include POCT for cardiac markers, infectious agents (eg, HIV, influenza A/B, respiratory syncytial virus), fetal fibronectin, platelet function, chemistry (eg, basic metabolic panel, lipid panel), and drugs of abuse. In some cases, established POCT technologies have found new applications that have significantly expanded their use. For example, bedside glucose testing was originally developed for routine inpatient diabetic monitoring. In recent years, these devices have been used for the management of tight glycemic control in acute care settings and to monitor premature infants for hypoglycemia in neonatal intensive care units. Finally, the menu of tests available on individual small bench-top or handheld devices has expanded. For example, devices are now available that can perform a number of routine chemistry tests, coagulation tests, and immunoassays on a single platform. Further expansion of the test menu and consolidation of devices to perform a larger number of tests will likely continue.

One important area of testing for which there are no practical point-of-care options is the complete blood count. The complete blood count is often required along with various chemistry tests to complete the laboratory assessment in both inpatient and outpatient settings. Although instruments are available that could be used at the point-of-care, these devices are basically scaled-down laboratory instruments that are impractical for use in most POCT applications.

Another important development is the expansion of POCT into the over-the-counter consumer market. This process is similar to that of the over-the-counter pharmaceutical market. Many drugs have been approved for sale directly to patients without a prescription and the list continues to grow. Patients can also purchase some types of monitoring devices, such as blood pressure meters and thermometers. The emergence of home testing had its origins when technologies were first developed to allow diabetics to monitor their blood sugar values using simple handheld glucose meters. Examples of other types of home testing include meters to monitor anticoagulation, urine pregnancy tests, fertility tests, cholesterol measuring devices, and drugs-of-abuse tests. In a manner analogous to the over-the-counter pharmaceutical market, the trend towards home testing will likely continue to expand, reflecting a greater awareness of consumerism in the laboratory testing market.

As a result of advances in technology and of the complex, ever-evolving, regulatory requirements, POCT has become recognized as an established subspecialty within the field of laboratory medicine. A number of textbooks in laboratory medicine contain chapters dedicated to POCT.[4,5] In many regions, professional organizations have been established with a focus on the interests of medical professionals involved in POCT. Several textbooks have been published on POCT, including books by Kost,[6] Price and Hicks,[7] and Nichols.[8] The American Association for Clinical Chemistry (AACC) has an established Critical Care/Point-of-Care Division with an affiliated journal, *Point-of-Care: The Journal of Near Patient Testing Technology*. Recently, the AACC established a certification program for point-of-care coordinators. The emergence of POCT as a subspecialty will likely continue.

UTILITY OF POCT

POCT may be used in a variety of applications:[1]

Screening: fecal occult blood, cholesterol, capillary blood glucose testing for diabetic screening at health fairs

Diagnosis: pregnancy testing, cardiac markers, rapid strep A testing

Medical management: bedside glucose, gastric occult blood, blood gases, electrolytes, activated clotting time

Patient management: cardiac markers used to triage patients to an observation unit versus an inpatient medical unit; urine pregnancy screen as a preradiology test in a trauma unit

Home use: patient self-monitoring–capillary glucose testing, ovulation testing, home coagulation monitoring

Medical management refers to testing for managing a clinical condition, such as bedside capillary glucose testing to maintain glycemic control in diabetic patients. In contrast, management of patients refers to testing performed to assist in managing the patient within the hospital. For example, cardiac markers may be used in conjunction with clinical data to triage patients to one of several different types of hospital beds, such as an observation unit, a general medical unit, or an intensive care setting. The decision is primarily related to hospital operations with the aim being to place the patient in the most cost-effective and clinically appropriate setting. In all of these applications, the key to the selection of POCT versus the central laboratory is the priority of rapid turnaround time over other considerations. The utility of POCT is on one level conceptual, and on another level based on evidence published in the medical literature. Since publication of the first *Clinics* issue on this topic, a number of peer-reviewed studies have been published documenting improved clinical outcomes and, more commonly, improved efficiency of clinical operations. These studies are described in more detail in a subsequent article.

A LOOK TO THE FUTURE

In the previous issue of *Clinics In Laboratory Medicine* in 2001, the following predictions were made.

Shifting of care to the home setting: Many laboratory tests are now available for home use, including an expanding menu of over-the-counter test kits available at the retail level to the general public. The expansion of home testing reflects a greater level of independence of the consumer from the traditional medical establishment. It is now possible for patients to evaluate their own testing needs, to select a technology at competitive prices, and to perform and interpret their own test results without the aid of a medical professional. This situation is analogous to over-the-counter pharmaceuticals that do not require a prescription.

Comment: As outlined in a subsequent article, penetration of POCT into the home has continued to expand. In addition to capillary blood glucose testing, self-monitoring of anticoagulation is now an accepted alternative to achieve reliable management of coumadin therapy. Many new tests are now available in over-the-counter formats and this trend will likely continue.

Recognition of the importance of integrated patient management and the impact of laboratory turnaround time on the total cost of care: This concept contrasts to the approach of looking only at the unit cost of laboratory tests versus POCT. Traditionally, financial evaluations of laboratories have been based on the cost per reportable test result. This perspective fails to consider the impact of the laboratory on other clinical services. The contribution of the laboratory to the total cost of care is difficult to measure. Consequently, it is easy to understand the preference of administrators for cost comparisons that can be readily measured. The laboratory has not generally been appreciated as an enabling technology that can facilitate (or impair) the delivery of care. In an era where patient length of stay in the hospital is perceived as critical to financial success, low unit cost at the expense of long turnaround time is decidedly counterproductive.

Comment: Many hospitals in the United States are facing capacity restraints. Frequently, all emergency room and inpatient beds are full. Other services, such as radiology, operate on extended hours, sometimes scheduling patients into the night. In some cases, POCT has been shown to decrease emergency room or hospital length of stay. Rapid whole-blood creatinine testing has been implemented in a number of radiology departments to screen patients for kidney disease. This testing assists in prevention of contrast-induced acute kidney damage and permits efficient patient flow, avoiding the need to wait for a creatinine measurement from the central laboratory. It is likely that other applications of POCT will be shown to improve clinical operations and assist in the management of hospital capacity.

Multitasked workers: New staffing models on patient units have focused on developing nursing assistants and multitasked workers. Hospitals continue to reevaluate the skill sets of workers with an emphasis on reducing the number of hospital workers that interact with the patient. For example, many institutions have transferred phlebotomy from the laboratory to unit-based nursing assistants. These new multitasked clinical assistants create opportunities to deploy POCT in areas that in the past may not have been feasible.

Comment: This trend was common in the late 1990s and is now firmly established in many hospitals. The ability of "multitasked workers" to perform an increasing variety of POCT has not been as robust as I predicted back in 2001. There are many reasons for this, including, perhaps, enforcement of increasingly complex regulatory requirements, expansion in nontesting-related duties for these workers, and the lack of user-friendly, foolproof POCT devices that can perform clinically relevant tests linked to a robust POCT data management system. Until POCT becomes essentially error-free both in terms of specimen analysis and data connectivity, it is unlikely that a major expansion of POCT will occur on hospital inpatient units. A possible exception is blood gas and electrolyte testing in acute care settings where POCT is increasingly the norm.

Critical labor shortages for medical technologists in the United States: During the 1990s, many schools of medical technology either closed or reduced their class sizes, creating an inevitable severe shortage of skilled medical technologists. Consequently, many laboratories do not have adequate staff to perform an ever-increasing volume of tests from an expanding test menu, and to respond to demand for more rapid turnaround time. With a national shortage of medical technologists continuing to worsen, there is little hope that this situation will change soon. POCT presents one option for the hospital when essential services cannot be provided by the central laboratory.

Comment: The shortage of medical technologists and the lack of sufficient training programs has not changed over the past 8 years. In many cases, laboratories have unfilled vacancies and cannot recruit qualified technologists. Yet, in most institutions, the volume and complexity of testing has been steadily increasing. One solution is to automate the central laboratory. Indeed many hospitals have already installed highly automated production lines to manage high-volume testing. However, it is common that a clinical service will require rapid testing to improve the efficiency of patient care.

The central laboratory may frequently be incapable of meeting this demand and, as a result, POCT is an increasingly viable option.

Considering the trends described above, the question inevitably arises: What is the future of POCT circa 2009 in both the short and long term? I am often asked this question and I am reminded of a quote from Yogi Berra: "It's difficult to make predictions, especially about the future." With that caveat, I will attempt to look into the future. This discussion will focus on the American situation, with which I am most familiar. Future trends in other countries, both industrialized and developing, may be quite different. To answer the question, it is important to consider some of the major trends that may affect POCT positively or negatively (**Box 4**). On one end of the spectrum, it could be projected that advances in technology and the need for rapid turnaround time will drive the exponential expansion of POCT. This scenario assumes the emergence of a catalyst that changes the paradigm of laboratory services, such as the development of (1) new devices capable of performing a broad menu of tests on a single portable POCT platform, including routine chemistries and hematology; or (2) a significant number of new tests that are most appropriately performed at the point-of-care and are required for medical reasons or to improve the efficiency of hospital/outpatient operations (eg, molecular-based POCT diagnostics for infectious disease).

In this scenario, POCT would realize significant and sustained rate of growth above, or at the expense of, that of central laboratories. In the most extreme case, nurses could provide most of the high-volume routine tests (chemistry, hematology) at the point-of-care using handheld or bedside devices. A similar situation could occur in outpatient sites. However, a device capable of performing this expanded menu of tests is some years away. Of note it is not sufficient for the device to perform most, but not all, of the routine tests because a second sample would still need to be sent to the laboratory thus diminishing the advantage of the POCT approach.

On the opposite extreme, the use of POCT could fall because of such factors as high unit cost, overregulation, or a demonstrated failure of these technologies to drive improvements in patient care or operational efficiency. Given the high cost of health care in the United States, it is reasonable to expect significant pressure to reduce costs by Medicare and third-party payers. Given that POCT is generally more expensive on a unit-cost basis than centralized testing, it will be tempting for hospitals needing to reduce operating budgets and having difficulty complying with regulations to eliminate all but the most essential POCT. Furthermore, the true advantages of

---

Box 4
Some factors that may affect the future of POCT

Increased regulation

Cost considerations

Reimbursement issues

New and consolidated instruments

Expanded test menu

Medical necessity for rapid turnaround time

Efforts to increase efficiency of hospital/outpatient operations

Shortages of medical technologists

Demand for home self-testing

POCT in terms of improving medical outcomes or operational efficiency have only occasionally been demonstrated in the medical literature.

Between these two extremes and perhaps the more likely scenario is the prospect that the menu and test volume of both POCT and central laboratory testing will continue to grow. Indeed, this has been the case over at least the past decade. The population of the United States is growing and continues to age. These trends will create more demand for laboratory services. Increasing pressure to improve hospital operations and patient outcomes will result in new niches for POCT (eg, creatinine in radiology).

In conclusion, the status of POCT will for the foreseeable future be driven by many of the same factors that affect clinical laboratories. Increased volume and expansion of the test menu will be moderated by the requirement for regulatory compliance, the pressure to control cost, and the need to demonstrate clear benefits of POCT over central laboratory testing. It is my hope that at some point in the future, a third issue on this topic will chronicle how these many factors affected the development of POCT and ultimately clinical care.

REFERENCES

1. Lewandrowski K, guest editor. Point of care testing. Clinics in Laboratory Medicine, Vol. 21 number 2. St. Louis (MO): Elsevier Saunders; 2001.
2. Lewandrowski K, Cheek R, Nathan N, et al. Implementation of capillary blood glucose monitoring in a teaching hospital and determination of program requirements to maintain quality testing. Am J Med 1992;93:419–26.
3. Lewandrowski K. Harming patients with quality: a commentary concerning the opportunity cost of excessive regulation. Point of care 2005;4:142–5.
4. Price C, St John A. Point of care testing (chapter 12). In: Burtis C, Ashwood E, Bruns D, editors. Tietz textbook of clinical chemistry and molecular diagnostics. 4th edition. St Louis (MO): Elsevier Saunders; 2006.
5. Threatte G. Point of care and physician office testing (chapter 6). In: McPherson R, Pincus M, editors. Henry's clinical diagnosis and management by laboratory methods. 21st edition. St Louis (MO): Elsevier Saunders; 2007.
6. Kost GJ, editor. Principles and practice of point-of-care testing. 1st edition. Philadelphia (PA): Lippincott Williams and Wilkins; 2002.
7. Price C, Hicks J, editor. Point of care testing. 1st edition. Washington (DC): AACC Press; 1999.
8. Nichols J, editor. Point-of-care testing: performance improvement and evidence-based outcomes. 1st edition. United Kingdom: Informa HealthCare; 2002.

Management of a Point-of-Care Testing Program

Kim Gregory, MT(ASCP), NCA, CLS, Kent Lewandrowski, MD*

KEYWORDS

- Point-of-care testing • Laboratory management
- Data management • Connectivity• Regulatory compliance

Point-of-care testing (POCT) has grown at an average rate of 9% percent per year over the last 8 years.[1] At the same time issues concerning the management of a POCT program have continued to be problematic. The perception of improved operational efficiencies or outcomes for patients when rapid POCT is employed often takes precedence over the difficulties encountered with regulatory compliance, quality assurance, and cost. The management of a POCT program has been outlined in the first edition of *Clinics in Laboratory Medicine: Point-of-Care Testing* and in books on POCT that have been previously published.[2–6] The goal of this article is to update the reader on contemporary topics in the management of POCT.

Highlights of the discussion on POCT management from the first edition of *Clinics in Laboratory Medicine* published in 2001 included the following key points as described by Lewandrowski[3] in the articled entitled "Point-of-care testing: an overview and a look to the future":

> Traditionally, POCT was unregulated and little effort was made by hospitals to establish an approach to managing these technologies. Predictably, issues concerning the quality of test results became apparent, resulting in the establishment of regulatory requirements that have been enforced by hospital accreditation organizations. Failure to comply with regulatory mandates may have major consequences. The need to address regulatory requirements combined with rapid expansion of POCT technologies has resulted in a concerted effort by institutions to manage POCT as a formal hospital program.

The first step in developing a strategy to manage POCT involves setting up an interdisciplinary POC management team, including the laboratory, physicians, and nurses. The POC team has the responsibility of determining the test menu, selecting

---

This article was adapted in part from the author's chapter in the forthcoming *Clinics in Laboratory Medicine* Point-of-Care Testing

Department of Pathology, Massachusetts General Hospital, Gray 5 Chemistry, Fruit St, Boston, MA 02114, USA

* Corresponding author.

E-mail address: klewandrowski@partners.org (K. Lewandrowski).

Clin Lab Med 29 (2009) 433–448
doi:10.1016/j.cll.2009.06.006
0272-2712/09/$ – see front matter © 2009 Elsevier Inc. All rights reserved.

technologies, establishing policies and procedures, ensuring training and regulatory compliance, and providing advisory assistance to the end users of POC technologies.

Efforts to organize a POCT program in the authors' institution have evolved over the years. In 1990, we became aware of the existence of bedside glucose testing being performed in the hospital. The clinical laboratories were asked to design and implement a quality control/quality assurance program. Our early experiences with bedside glucose testing have been previously reported. In 1992, we turned over management of the POC program to the Department of Nursing. The clinical laboratories maintained an advisory and consultative role with the Department of Nursing, which was responsible for ongoing quality assurance activities. During 1996, it became apparent that this approach was inadequate to maintain appropriate quality standards. Furthermore, POCT was expanding to include other tests in addition to bedside glucose testing. This expansion led us to redefine our strategy for the management of POCT. The first step was to organize an interdisciplinary POC team composed of representatives from the clinical laboratories, the Department of Nursing, and administration (**Fig. 1**). The POC team was assigned responsibility and authority for managing the POC program and for implementing continuous quality improvement efforts. To ensure that the POC team had sufficient authority to implement major objectives, a steering committee was established that meets quarterly. The steering committee includes the Chief of Pathology, the Director of Clinical Laboratories, the director of the POC program, laboratory administration, the Associate Director of Nursing, the Chief Medical Officer, and the Senior Vice President for Ancillary Services. The POC team reports to the steering committee and develops and implements initiatives that have been approved by the steering committee. The POC team is composed of a clinical pathologist medical director, a representative from laboratory administration, a medical technologist dedicated to POC, and a nursing POC coordinator. In 2001 the management team used 1.72 full-time equivalent (FTE) personnel with a total annual cost of $96,509. Day-to-day management of the POC program is the responsibility of unit-based nurse managers who are responsible for compliance with regulatory and institutional policies. Labor cost estimates for the time spent by unit-based nurse managers are not included in the estimate listed above.

The next step in organizing the program was to perform an institution-wide survey to determine what tests were being performed at the POC. The audit was performed by mailing survey forms to all nursing units and by site visits and interviews with the unit nurse managers. In a number of cases, tests were identified that the unit managers did not consider to fall under the definition of POCT. In addition to interviewing the nurse managers, we also inspected the nursing units. On several occasions, we discovered supplies and reagents for tests that were not reported by the unit.

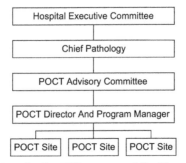

Fig. 1. Organizational structure for the POC program at the Massachusetts General Hospital.

The most commonly performed POC test at the authors' center is bedside glucose testing. Dipstick urinalysis and fecal occult blood testing are also commonly performed. In total in 2001, over 400,000 tests were performed at the POC, comprising 8.2% of all laboratory tests at the hospital.

The next step is to assess the medical need for each POC test and determine which technologies are most appropriate for the intended application. This assessment requires interviews with physicians or nurses and is best performed by the POCT medical director. Questions to be considered when assessing medical need include why the site is performing POCT, what turnaround time is required from a medical perspective and from the perspective of unit operations, and what analytic performance is acceptable for the intended application.

The next task is to develop policies and procedures. This task includes establishing a quality control and quality assurance program to ensure regulatory compliance and to maintain quality testing. A corrective action plan to remedy ongoing deficiencies is essential to the success of the program. In some cases, this may require mandates to discontinue testing in noncompliant sites. The corrective action plan is particularly important for manual POCT in which auditing of quality control and quality assurance activities is more difficult than for instrumented tests because of the necessity of maintaining manual records. In contrast, oversight of instrumented tests can be facilitated by electronic data management (DM) systems and requires less on-site assessment of compliance. The key to successful corrective action is to ensure that the POC team has the authority to make decisions concerning the suitability of testing at any given site. When a site is found to be noncompliant, an effort should be made to educate the personnel who are performing the test as to the necessary requirements for compliance with the program. If remedial action is not successful, consideration should be given to removing testing when compliance cannot be achieved with the quality assurance program. One recommendation to ensure the authority of the POCT management team is to have an institutional policy whereby the POCT team controls the Clinical Laboratory Improvement Amendment (CLIA) certificates for all testing sites.

Once a POCT program has been established, the team should begin a continuous process improvement effort designed to enhance the efficiency and ease of compliance with the program. This process requires ongoing site inspections and continuing education, and may involve implementing new technologies, consolidation of technologies, and, in some cases, elimination of POC tests that do not meet quality standards. For example, our site inspections revealed that several urinalysis dipstick products were being used in the hospital for a variety of applications. These tests included screening for hematuria and urine pH on oncology units, monitoring hydration status in pediatric patients and those with diabetes insipidus, and general urinalysis applications. Each product required its own policy and procedure and quality control, training, and competency assessment programs. First, the medical need for each type of test was examined to ensure that the application was appropriate and that the technologies performed at an acceptable level for the intended application. For example, pH paper to measure urine pH had not been validated and was eliminated. Owing to the availability of multiple products, maintaining compliance with the POC program was extremely difficult for users of urinalysis test strips because there were too many different products, standards for performance were not established, and some of the applications were inappropriate. The management decision was to consolidate all of these technologies to a single urinalysis strip and to establish one set of policies and procedures, training, and quality control. This change radically simplified the management of POC urinalysis testing in our institution.

As described previously, several problems and challenges encountered at the authors' center have led the hospital to continually modify and improve the approach to managing bedside testing technologies. Based on these experiences, the following observations deserve specific comment:

The management of a successful POCT program requires an interdepartmental team composed of the clinical laboratories, nursing, and hospital administration.

Identifying sites performing POCT and the menu of tests on each unit requires on-site interviews and inspections of individual units. Physical inspection of the facility may reveal testing that has not been disclosed by mailed surveys. On-site inspections also allow for relationships to be developed between the POC management team and the unit nurse managers. These relationships are critical when quality improvement initiatives are implemented.

It is important to interview physicians and nurses to understand the medical justi-fication for POCT. In some cases, the explanation for a particular test is well es-tablished (such as bedside glucose testing), whereas in other situations the medical justification may be unwarranted. Understanding the medical justifica-tion for POCT is necessary to assist in planning the POC program, in developing alternatives to POCT, and in implementing process improvements for tests that are to remain at the bedside.

In large institutions, quality assurance inspections are necessary to establish the baseline performance of the quality assurance program. On-site inspections are labor intensive and are insufficient to maintain the quality of the program. Over the long term, a growing POCT program may expand to include multiple technologies in a variety of applications. It is necessary to implement a contin-uous quality improvement effort to streamline workflow and enhance the quality of POCT.

A CONTEMPORARY PERSPECTIVE ON THE MANAGEMENT OF POCT (CIRCA 2009)

The previous text has outlined the state of POCT management circa 2001. Since that time, those of us who are responsible for managing POCT have gained new insights on how best to manage these technologies outside of the clinical laboratory. The following discussion highlights our more recent experiences at the Massachusetts General Hospital with an emphasis on contemporary issues in POCT management.

Structure of the POCT Program

The first step in organizing a POCT program is to decide which model will be used to manage the program. There are two basic approaches—centralized or decentralized. There is not a preferred structure. The choice of which model to use depends on several factors, such as the size of the institution, the number of testing sites, the test menu, the number of available POCT coordinators, the administrative structure of the institution, and the culture of the institution. Both management models benefit from the establishment of a multidisciplinary POCT committee. The committee should consist of members that represent all important aspects of the program, including clinicians, nurses, laboratorians, finance, information technology, and regulatory compliance. Usually, a pathologist is designated as the director of the POCT program and holds the CLIA certificate under his or her name.

The centralized model gives more control to the clinical laboratory. The laboratory controls the CLIA certificate and manages the program. Many smaller institutions delegate management of POCT to a medical technologist or quality assurance/safety officer who typically has other duties outside of POCT. In larger hospitals, it is desirable to designate a dedicated position (or team) exclusively to the POC program. Often, the amount of work required to manage a compliant program is underestimated, and additional resources may be required.

In the centralized model, the POCT team manages all aspects of the program including validation of devices, implementation of testing, training, DM, and quality assurance. An essential feature of the program is to give the POCT team the authority to discontinue testing at sites that fail to follow requirements for regulatory compliance.

The decentralized model delegates authority and responsibility to local site directors/coordinators who manage their own testing program. Usually, the laboratory serves in a consultative role to provide technical and regulatory expertise to support the individual sites. This approach gives the testing site a "hands-on" experience with testing and compliance; however, the decentralized model is more vulnerable to problems with regulatory compliance because individual sites may neglect to manage their compliance due to competing pressures for their time in managing the many day-to-day issues the site encounters.

At the authors' center, we have had an established POCT program that continues to resemble the description by Lewandrowski. As POCT has expanded in our institution, we have added more resources to the management team. In 1991 we deployed 1.72 FTE personnel to POCT management. In 2009 we now have 3.6 FTE personnel, including a 0.1 FTE medical director, 1 FTE administrative associate director, 2 FTE POCT coordinators, and a 0.5 FTE nursing POCT liaison. **Fig. 2** shows an organizational chart for the POCT program at our institution. We manage three types of CLIA certificates, including waived, moderate complexity (non-waived), and provider-performed microscopy (PPM). The largest testing site is patient care services, which includes all of the waived testing (bedside glucose testing, dipstick urinalysis, and fecal occult blood) performed by nurses on inpatient units. Several "special function laboratories" perform a variety of testing such as activated clotting time, blood gases, and microscopy. There are a number of off-site POCT locations. Each CLIA certificate is assigned to a physician or doctoral staff member, and each site has a local site director who is responsible for testing and compliance.

An important observation concerning **Fig. 2** is the size and scope of our POCT program. Since 2001 hospital sites have continued to expand into the surrounding community. With this expansion, the number of POCT sites has grown. Our program now encompasses not just the hospital campus itself but also a number of outpatient facilities in the Boston metropolitan area. Performing site inspections and keeping up to date with testing activities at off campus locations is both time consuming and challenging. It would be tempting to place too much reliance on e-mail communication to manage these sites. In our experience, this would be a major mistake. The importance of regular on-site inspections cannot be overemphasized. Inspections detect problems that have been overlooked by the testing sites and ensure that formerly compliant sites remain so. In addition, inspections permit the POCT team to build working relationships with the sites which are invaluable when issues are identified. A common problem encountered at sites that have historically been compliant is that turnover of staff at the site can result in rapid noncompliance when the key POCT person at the site is replaced.

Expansion of the POCT menu and an increase in the number of personnel dedicated to POCT management has been a consistent trend at many institutions across the country. As this trend appears likely to continue, we should expect further growth in testing and in POCT programs. Our POCT management team receives frequent

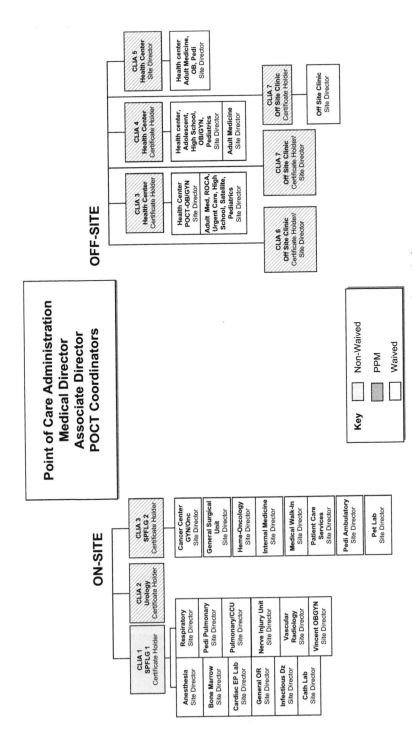

Fig. 2. POCT and affiliated laboratories organizational chart at the Massachusetts General Hospital.

requests from clinicians to expand the POCT menu or to add new POCT sites for existing technologies such as bedside glucose testing. All new POCT must be approved by the POCT management team. This process is formalized and is controlled by the fact that the laboratory holds the CLIA certificates for the entire institution. All sites wishing to implement new testing must submit a POCT request form as shown in **Fig. 3**. Based on this form, the team can assess the appropriateness of the testing and determine the programmatic requirements to maintain regulatory compliance. A generic description of the process for initiating new POCT is outlined below. One important caveat is that the requirements under CLIA are frequently supplemented with additional POCT regulatory requirements by the Joint Commission and the College of American Pathologists (CAP). An important role for the POCT management team is to stay current with changes in regulations, to inform nurses and physicians of these changes, and to assist in modifying the program to meet regulatory compliance. In large institutions with testing being performed in a number of locations, this task can be extremely challenging. It is essential for the POCT team to develop working relationships with the testing site directors and to have an effective mechanism for communication to all sites under their management.

GENERAL PROCESS FOR INITIATING NEW POCT

Most hospitals have had established POCT management programs for several years. These programs ensure regulatory compliance and manage the status quo testing activities. One of the most common issues we now face is a request from a clinical site to initiate new POCT. For this reason we outline our general approach to this common situation.

The first steps for any site wishing to perform POCT are to determine the test menu, find a qualified medical director, and apply for a CLIA certificate. CLIA certificates fall into three categories: certificates of waiver, PPM, and certificates of accreditation. Professional requirements for the person holding the CLIA certificate have changed in recent years.

The next step is to determine which accrediting agencies standards the program will follow. A stand-alone clinic or doctor's office may choose to follow the federal CLIA standards and those of the state Department of Public Health. These sites may be inspected by the Department of Public Health or another accreditation agency such as the Commission on Laboratory Accreditation. Sites affiliated with a hospital laboratory can choose to be accredited by the Joint Commission, or if their laboratory is CAP accredited, they may wish to accredit their POCT program with CAP.[7,8] Both agencies have advantages and disadvantages, and their regulatory requirements for POCT include requirements above the minimum standards mandated by CLIA. The decision is up to the medical director. In some cases the medical director may decide to divide up the test methods based on complexity between the two regulatory agencies. Implementation of the Joint Commission tracer inspection methodology in January 2006[7] has changed the approach the Joint Commission takes when inspecting POCT. Traditionally, POCT was inspected only during the laboratory survey; however, with the tracer method POCT can also be scrutinized during the hospital survey. In a hospital where the POCT program is CAP accredited, the Joint Commission may still review POCT sites during the hospital survey. Another major change arising from the tracer methodology is the manner in which the inspection is conducted. In the pre-tracer approach, the inspection largely consisted of reviews of documentation. This review was usually performed in a conference room, and the POCT team could exert some degree of control over the inspection process. With the new tracer method,

Patient Test Result/Quality Control Log :Rapid Strep A

Start a new log when opening a new box of 50 Test Sticks. Both the positive and negative external controls must be analyzed when opening a new box. Document the following three Internal Controls with every test (indicate with a check mark if controls are acceptable): **QC1:** Combining reagents 1&2 changes color from pink to yellow. **QC2:** Red line appears on stick in 5-10 minutes. **QC3:** Background in control line area is clear.

Kit Lot #:   Expiration Date: Internal Controls:

Date Collected	Time Collected	Patient Name	Patient Unit Number	Sample Result Pos or Neg	Pink to yellow?	Red line?	Bckgrnd clear?	Operator	Lab Result
		Positive Control	Abnormal						
		Negative Control	Normal						

Reviewed by: Date

Fig. 3. Sample log sheet for a manual visually read POC test.

most of the inspection is conducted in the care units themselves. Frequently, employees are interviewed about policies and procedures including the observation of actual testing. In this approach, the POCT team has much less control over how the inspection actually occurs. Most of the interactions with the inspectors occur between nurses and physicians rather than the POCT management team.

Before any new test can be implemented in clinical practice, the method needs to be validated. This task is usually performed by the POCT management team. The process includes assessment of diagnostic accuracy, precision, reportable range, normal reference values, quality control, interferences, and other analytical variables. The Clinical Laboratory Standards Institute (CLSI) has published general guidelines for performance of method validations.[9] In practice with some POC tests, ridged adherence to these guidelines may not be practical. For example, many single-use disposable POCT cartridges are expensive on a unit cost basis, making it cost prohibitive to perform extensive validation studies. Other POC tests such as fetal fibronectin or platelet function studies do not have an established predicate method in the laboratory to compare against. Usually, POC tests use whole blood samples which may produce different values from serum or plasma samples tested for the same analyte in the central laboratory. In some cases, seemingly trivial issues such as the type of anticoagulant required for the test (heparin, EDTA, citrate) will affect test results. It may be difficult to obtain whole blood samples with the required anticoagulant without the need to collect extra tubes of blood from patients, especially when the central laboratory method uses a different sample type from the POC method. Obtaining extra samples beyond that needed for clinical care requires patient informed consent. For these reasons, performing method validation studies on POC devices requires judgment and expertise. Frequently, the process involves pragmatic trade-offs that deviate from established method validation protocols.

A different situation occurs when an existing device is replaced or testing is set up with a new device at an additional site. In this case, the method has already been validated but it is still necessary to document that the new device is performing according to manufacturer's specifications. Usually, performance verification is straightforward and requires only a simplified protocol consisting of calibration verification and measurement of a limited number of quality control samples or patient specimens.

The final steps in the process of establishing a new POC test is implementation, followed by ongoing monitoring of quality and regulatory compliance under the umbrella of the POCT management program. Several issues need to be addressed during the implementation phase as shown in **Box 1**. Each of these components must be in place before patient testing can commence. Once the test is put into clinical practice, the task of ongoing management must be considered. Many of these issues are self-explanatory or were covered in the first edition of this issue; however, some require further comment based on new developments or additional experience as described below.

Training and Competency

Management of training and competency is no simple task, regardless of the number of staff involved. In large institutions, the number of personnel to be trained may number in the thousands. Turnover of employees increases the challenge of tracking initial training, 6-month competency review (if required), and annual competency. One approach to accomplishing this task is to embed the required training into the employee's initial orientation and annual performance review. The training data can then be assembled in an electronic database to track the status of each employee's training

---

Box 1
Issues to address when implementing a new POC test

Method validation

Policy and procedure manual

Staff training

Clear definition of the roles and responsibilities of site personnel and the POC management team

Mechanism for documentation of patient test results and for documentation of data required for regulatory compliance

Supplies and inventory management

Defined quality control and quality assurance program

Mechanism for ongoing monitoring of testing

---

certification. Recent CLIA guidelines now require physicians to undergo initial training and annual competency assessment. Some hospitals use the physician credentialing process to maintain up to date physician training for waived tests; however, the frequency of recredentialing (typically every 2 years) may not be sufficient to achieve compliance with the annual competency assessment requirement for PPM.

Regulatory agencies now mandate two forms of competency for most testing (excluding PPM performed by physicians). **Box 2** illustrates the requirements. The requirement for two forms of competency assessment has significantly complicated training and documentation activities. In a typical large hospital, several thousand staff require annual competency assessment; therefore, the effort including the actual training and its documentation has essentially doubled.

Box 2
Competency assessment guidelines of the College of American Pathologists (CAP) and the Joint Commission

Joint Commission

Written quiz

Direct observation

Quality control performance

Successful proficiency survey

Testing blind specimens

College of American Pathologists (CAP) (see POCT)

Written quiz

Direct observation of routine patient test performance

Quality control performance

Successful proficiency survey

Monitoring the recording and reporting of test results

Review of intermediate test results or worksheets, quality control records, and so on

Evaluation of problem-solving skills

Elements to be included in a training program have remained the same since their description in 1999 by Burnett.[10] **Box 3** summarizes the training elements required for proper performance of testing.

Initial training with hands-on exposure continues to be the most effective form of training on new methods. Many POCT programs use the vendor to provide initial training. So-called "train the trainer" classes develop expert operators who can provide expertise post installation. Larger installations may require 24 × 7 training of all staff. Ongoing training is maintained by the POCT management team, designated site trainers, or clinical educators in the Department of Nursing.

Regulatory agencies mandate two forms of competency for most testing performed. **Box 2** illustrates examples of the requirements. Ongoing competency is often documented at the employee annual performance. To improve efficiency, many institutions have moved their competency programs online. Several programs are available, such as Healthstream, ePRO, or www.medtraining.org. Medtraining has the advantage of providing content from a laboratory perspective; however, an enterprise system such as Healthstream may be more effective due to the support of the Department of Nursing.

One should consider the information technology infrastructure of the site when choosing or creating content. Lack of sound cards (due to patient noise-satisfaction concerns), locked down clinical software builds that prevent drivers such as Active X from downloading, and institutional restrictions on Internet access may create significant problems for the training program. For example, at the authors' center, the POCT team worked with laboratory information system (LIS) training staff to create an introductory video for clinicians about changes in our new glucose meter. A narrated video was created in Adobe Captivate; however, the clinical computer builds on our units did

---

Box 3
Training for correct performance of testing

Awareness of pre-analytical factors

Obtaining the correct specimen

Importance of clinical contraindications

Sample handling and labeling (if applicable)

Stability of sample

Stability of reagents, test strips, test devices

Demonstrable expertise in analytical skills

Operation, calibration, and routine maintenance, understanding of analytical limitations of the instrument

Recognition of potential instrument or test system malfunction and simple trouble-shooting techniques

Principles, procedures, and documentation of internal quality control and external quality assessment

Understanding of proper documentation of patient results including connectivity requirements

Cleaning, decontamination, and disposal procedures

Data from Burnett D. Training and certification. In: Price C, Hicks J. Point-of-care testing. Washington (DC): AACC Press; 1999.

not have sound cards. To solve the problem, closed captioning was added, and the video was also translated into Spanish. The video worked perfectly on the computers of the POCT staff but did not work on the clinical computer builds on the units due to security restrictions. We were unable to overcome the obstacle, and the video remains unused.

Documentation and Data Management Connectivity

Considerable attention has been directed to development of the electronic medical record (EMR). President Barack Obama as one of his many initiatives to lower health care costs has advocated significant investment in electronic medical information technology.[11] The intention is to invest $10 billion a year over the next 5 years in an effort to move the US health care system to broad adoption of standards-based electronic health information systems, including EMRs.[11] Many other industries have comprehensive electronic systems, but health care information technology has lagged behind. For example, data released in 2009 indicate that only a fraction of hospitals have an EMR in place.

There are many challenges to transitioning to EMRs. No single system accommodates all essential functions. Changing the culture of physicians and nurses to switch to electronic documentation may be difficult. Connectivity for POCT has advanced considerably over the past 2 decades. Glucose meters were the front leaders in device connectivity. Meters are returned to docking stations that are connected by serial or data port connections to a DM system that can be interfaced to the LIS. More advanced systems have an admission, discharge, and transfer (ADT) feed connected to the DM system. Although some systems can send the ADT feed directly to the meter (which provides the staff with two patient identifier confirmations), not every POCT device has this functionality.

Challenges with connectivity include proper planning for installation (eg, power sources, data jack availability) and ongoing troubleshooting of station outages (eg, disconnected data cables or power sources). The more complicated the infrastructure of the hospital, the more difficult it is to troubleshoot connectivity problems which may arise in either the hardware or software.

In 2001 the Connectivity Industry Consortium (CIC) achieved its goal to develop a standard for POC connectivity based on existing IEEE and HL7 standards and on specifications developed by the CIC. The guidelines were published by the CLSI [formerly the National Committee for Clinical Laboratory Standards (NCCLS)] in 2002 and targeted medical device manufacturers. The CLSI updated the guidelines for health care providers in May of 2008 with publication of the POCT02-A.[12] Vendors now have a set of guidelines by which to develop connectivity friendly devices; however, in most situations, the connectivity solution is still not at the ideal of "plug and play" devices.

An institution installing a DM system for the first time should consider the infrastructure it wishes to support before purchasing a system. Security protocols and hardware requirements of the server must meet or exceed the requirements of the institution's information technology department.

There are two main models of DM systems and many hybrids in the marketplace in 2009. A vendor-neutral DM system (eg, RALS Plus by Medical Automation Systems, Inc, Charlottesville, VA) connects many devices from different vendors through one platform. The other option is an interface engine (eg, Telcor QML by Telcor, Lincoln, NE) that connects multiple vendors' DM software to the LIS. There are disadvantages to both systems.

With use of an integrated DM system, one is limited to the devices from vendors that the company has a relationship with. This relationship may result in a limitation in technology for the institution. An interface engine may work with all vendors; however, this system is not fully bidirectional. The POCT coordinator is forced to be proficient with multiple vendor-supplied DM systems to configure the equipment. This setup may require multiple operator databases (a cumbersome task regardless of the number of operators).

An ADT interface feed should be connected to the main DM system that interfaces to the LIS. It is prudent to consider maintenance of only one ADT interface. Vendors may advocate connecting the ADT feed to their proprietary systems; however, updating and making changes to multiple interfaces can be time consuming.

Wireless connectivity in the context of cell phone quality data transmission does not yet truly exist for POCT, although some pseudo-wireless solutions are available. Serial connections through personal computers often require a service to run in the background for data transmission. This setup can create various problems depending on the system and the personal computer's resources.

Network connections for each device are ideal; however, the availability of data jacks and power outlets can be limited even in ideal environments. Should one use a static or Dynamic Host Configuration Protocol (DHCP) IP address? Neither is plug and play; therefore, the decision comes down to the connectivity solution and the requirements of the information technology department. Some DM systems require input of the IP address in order to facilitate communication. DHCP addresses cause problems with this because they can change frequently, depending on the network settings. If allowed, giving an IP address a permanent lease will minimize disruptions. Clearly, in the current POCT environment, it is essential to have the full support of the information technology department to operate and maintain the POCT connectivity system. Regardless of the connectivity solution that is selected, many POC tests continue to be visually read, manually performed tests that will continue to require manual test records as shown in **Fig. 3**.

Quality Assurance and Compliance

Achieving satisfactory compliance with regulatory requirements is an essential component of a POC program. Compliance is a necessary foundation for ongoing quality assurance, but compliance alone is insufficient. Key features of the compliance program include the following:

- An interdisciplinary POCT management team with representatives from the laboratory, nursing, physicians, information systems, and hospital administration
- Clear delineation of authority from the institution for the POC team to administer the program
- Sufficient support from hospital information technology staff to implement, maintain, and improve POCT electronic DM systems
- Leadership for the POC team by a medical director and a senior administrative director
- Adequate staffing of the POC team with sufficient POC coordinators to oversee the program
- Clear written policies and procedures available to all testing sites
- Reliable and documented training and competency assessment program
- Electronic communication system (e-mail) to all sites
- Assignment of site directors to ensure local oversight and accountability

Systematic and frequent on-site inspections of testing sites to audit records and observe the testing environment

Frequent ongoing education of staff at POCT sites

Robust and proactive quality assurance and quality improvement program for POCT

Quality improvement requires a committed and ongoing effort by the POC leadership team to seek out opportunities to improve processes and enhance the value of POCT to clinicians caring for patients. A typical example would be a quality improvement initiative aimed at implementing a new POC test or an institutional effort to install an enterprise POCT DM system. Another more mundane example was described for consolidating dipstick urinalysis testing earlier in this article.

BILLING FOR POCT

Billing for POCT may occur in several locations, such as the physician's office, hospital-affiliated outpatient clinics, and inhospital inpatient units. Each of these settings presents unique challenges.

Physician's Offices

Before most private physician's offices will consider performing a POCT, it is usually mandatory that the test be reimbursable by Medicare and by third-party payers. The practice must purchase the supplies and incur labor expenses to perform the testing. These costs must be reimbursed to avoid financial loss to the practice. Not all POC tests are reimbursed by payors; in other cases, the reimbursed rate is not sufficient to cover the cost of testing. In many other situations, the reimbursed rate exceeds the cost, and the practice can make money by performing testing on site. This fact was one of the reasons why numerous practices in the past set up physician office laboratories (POLs) to perform testing on site. The POL market is a niche cottage industry, and several vendors make small bench top devices for performing common laboratory tests. These devices are one form of POCT. Additionally, conventional POC tests, such as rapid streptococcus A, influenza A/B, fecal occult blood, and urine pregnancy testing, are common and suitable products for POLs. Most practices use commercial billing companies to assist them in efficient collection of reimbursements.

Hospital-affiliated Outpatient Clinics

These practices are similar to the physician's office described previously, with the exception that they may be required to use the central hospital laboratory. POC tests may be performed and billed, but, typically, the menu of test options is more restricted. On a large hospital campus, the available revenue for billing for POCT can be substantial. The difficulty comes in getting the billing data into a suitable electronic format, especially with manually performed tests. Manual billing is cumbersome and incurs significant expense which may negate the revenues achieved from actual reimbursement.

Hospital Inpatients

In contrast to outpatient settings, reimbursement for testing performed on inpatients is usually rolled up into a single payment for the hospital event (diagnostic related group). The hospital gets paid a flat rate for the entire episode of care regardless of how many tests are performed or not performed. The incentive is to control excess utilization and avoid unnecessary testing. Hospital billing systems can capture and bill for POC tests at some preset fee schedule, creating "pseudo-revenue" in the budget, but in most cases this revenue is never actually collected. For this reason, many hospitals have made little effort to bill for POCT because setting up the billing system incurs cost but little actual revenue can be collected. Exceptions include self-pay patients and a limited number of indemnity insurance plans. Interestingly, some hospitals have used POCT billing data as an indirect means to audit test volume and utilization. When POCT is performed, especially manual tests, it can be difficult to determine who is doing the testing and at what volume.

HEALTH INSURANCE PORTABILITY AND ACCOUNTABILITY ACT

The Health Insurance Portability and Accountability Act (HIPAA) was passed in 1996 and required full implementation with all statutes by May of 2008. Failure to comply with HIPAA carries heavy civil and criminal penalties. The Business Associate Agreement (BAA) was implemented by health care institutions (covered entities) and private companies (business associates) to ensure compliance with Protected Health Information (PHI) and Electronic Protected Health Information. POCT devices and connectivity systems can easily be excluded from this process. It is important that the POCT program include BAAs either in the initial contract signed in purchasing or have all vendors sign a BAA and submit the document to the legal department. Broken devices are returned to vendors with PHI in their memory, and connectivity systems provide dial-in customer support that gives them access to PHI.

SUMMARY

The approach to managing a POCT program has evolved over recent years. Although many of the essential features of early POCT management programs remain intact, contemporary challenges including expansion of the test menu, changing regulatory requirements, and the development of more sophisticated DM connectivity requiring ongoing adaptation of POCT management programs. Despite significant improvements in test quality and regulatory compliance, significant challenges for the management of POCT will continue for the foreseeable future.

REFERENCES

1. Cambridge Consultants. Point-of-care: the demise of high throughput screening? Cambridge, England: Cambridge Consultants; 2006. p. 1–9.
2. Humbertson S. Management of a point-of-care program: organization, quality assurance and data management. Clin Lab Med 2001;21:255–68.
3. Lee-Lewandrowski E, Lewandrowski K. Point-of-care testing: an overview and a look to the future. Clin Lab Med 2001;21:217–40.
4. Kost GJ, editor. Principles and practice of point-of-care testing. 1st edition. Philadelphia: Lippincott Williams and Wilkins; 2002.
5. Price C, Hicks J, editors. Point of care testing. 1st edition. Washington (DC): AACC Press; 1999.
6. Nichols J, editor. Point-of-care testing: performance improvement and evidence-based outcomes. 1st edition. New York: Informa HealthCare; 2002.
7. The Joint Commission. Available at: http://www.jointcommission.org/AccreditationPrograms/Hospitals/AccreditationProcess/Tracer_Methodology.htm. Accessed April 27, 2009.
8. College of American Pathologists (CAP). Available at: www.CAP.org. Accessed April 27, 2009.

9. Krouwer J, Tholen D, Garber C, et al. Method comparison and bias estimation using patient samples: approved guideline, Vol. 22, No. 19. Wayne (PA): Clinical and Laboratory Standards Institute; 2002.

10. Burnett D. Training and certification. In: Price C, Hicks J, editors. Point-of-care testing. Washington (DC): AACC Press; 1999.

11. President Barack Obama. Available at: http://www.whitehouse.gov/agenda/technology/. Accessed April 27, 2009.

12. Implementation guide of POCT01 for health care providers. Available at: www.clsi.org. Accessed April 27, 2009.

Point-of-Care Testing Informatics

Ji Yeon Kim, MD, MPH[a], Kent Lewandrowski, MD[b],*

KEYWORDS

- Point-of-care • Informatics • Data management • Connectivity
- Electronic medical record • POCT1-A

Point-of-care testing (POCT) devices promise rapid "on-site" availability of an expanding menu of tests in locations outside the central laboratory, including at the patient's bedside.[1] Early POCT devices were located in such settings as the intensive care unit, where clinicians needed to monitor acute laboratory changes,[2] or on general inpatient medical units, where clinicians managed diabetic patients using bedside capillary glucose testing. Currently, POCT devices are popular for both acute and chronic patient management. However, while technologic advances have allowed for device miniaturization, ease of use, and increased test sophistication and accuracy, poor planning for data management connectivity and device software interoperability has limited integration of test results with the laboratory information system (LIS) and/or hospital information system (HIS). This has meant that, apart from the clinician who views the results at the time of testing, POCT results may not be available to other care providers and may be excluded from the patient's permanent medical record. Until issues concerning POCT data management and connectivity are adequately addressed, it is likely that continued expansion of POCT will be significantly impaired.

POINT-OF-CARE (POC) DATA MANAGEMENT: A HISTORICAL PERSPECTIVE

In the early 1990s, electronic data management for POCT was essentially nonexistent. With the relatively small number of devices, test results and quality control data were maintained using handwritten records. In many cases, the records were poorly maintained and impossible to audit.

As POCT became more widespread, laboratory accreditation agencies began more rigorous enforcement of regulations under the 1988 Clinical Laboratories

[a] Department of Pathology, Massachusetts General Hospital and Harvard Medical School, Pathology Service, WRN 219, Massachusetts General Hospital, 55 Fruit Street, Boston, MA 02114, USA
[b] Department of Pathology, Massachusetts General Hospital and Harvard Medical School, Gray 5-536 Chemistry, 55 Fruit Street, Boston, MA 02114, USA
* Corresponding author. Gray 5-536 Chemistry, Massachusetts General Hospital, 55 Fruit Street, Boston, MA 02114.
E-mail address: klewandrowski@partners.org (K. Lewandrowski).

Clin Lab Med 29 (2009) 449–461
doi:10.1016/j.cll.2009.06.014
0272-2712/09/$ – see front matter © 2009 Elsevier Inc. All rights reserved.

Improvement Amendments (CLIA). This development compelled manufacturers to develop technologies to better manage POCT data. The first systems were developed to support bedside glucose testing. These "first-generation" systems consisted of a laptop computer with rudimentary data management software. The laptop had to be carried to testing sites to download the data (**Table 1** and **Fig. 1**). The data was not interfaced to the LIS and presented only a historical archive of past testing activity.

"Second-generation" systems were also initially developed to support bedside glucose testing (**Fig. 2**). These systems employed a centralized desktop computer connected via the Ethernet to instrument docking stations located on the patient care units. When the device was placed into the docking station, stored data would be downloaded to the central data management system. The test data could then be transferred to the LIS/HIS using a computer interface. These systems permitted test data to become part of the patient's electronic medical record (EMR).

Even so, many hospitals to this day do not include most of the POCT patient data in the EMR. Like data in first-generation systems, the data was essentially historical, albeit closer to real time than when using a portable laptop system. Second-generation data managers were vendor-specific, closed architecture systems not designed to accommodate instruments from other manufacturers. Consequently, if several different POCT devices were used, multiple standalone data management systems were required.

Table 1	
Evolution of point-of-care data management systems	
Approach	**Comments**
Manual records	Unreliable and difficult to maintain; cannot be easily audited; originally used for all POCT; continues to be used extensively for manual visually read tests and low-volume instrumented tests where the cost of interfacing the instrument is excessive.
First generation (**Fig. 1**)	Used laptop computer that had to be carried to testing sites to download data; usually no interface to LIS or HIS; provided only historical testing and quality control data; systems could only interface to a single device type from one manufacturer.
Second generation (**Fig. 2**)	Central desktop computer connected by Ethernet to peripheral docking stations on patient care units; provides more frequent access to patient data at time of instrument docking or data transfer; bidirectional capability allows central data manager to communicate data to peripheral devices; could be interfaced to LIS and HIS; could not be interfaced to devices from more than one manufacturer.
Third generation (**Fig. 3**)	Similar to second generation but allows multivendor connectivity providing enterprise level data management solution.
Possible future data management system (**Fig. 4**)	Multivendor wireless connectivity using a single data management system with bidirectional communication to wireless-enabled POCT devices.

POCT devices downloaded to laptop (once a month) where information is aggregated

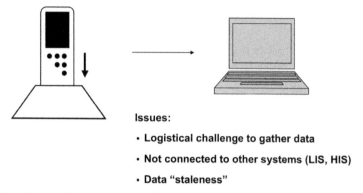

Issues:

- **Logistical challenge to gather data**
- **Not connected to other systems (LIS, HIS)**
- **Data "staleness"**

Fig. 1. Evolution of POCT connectivity, first generation.

"Third-generation" systems are now available that can accept data from multiple devices (**Fig. 3**). This single data management system can be interfaced to the LIS/HIS to provide true multivendor connectivity. Most hospitals in the United States currently employ one of these third-generation systems. However, as in the past, many hospitals continue to transmit only a fraction of POCT data into the EMR. Often the POCT data is stored in the data management system. The data is available for quality assurance audits and to document regulatory compliance, but never gets transmitted to the LIS or HIS. An ideal future "fourth-generation" system will employ bidirectional wireless technology to transmit data in real time to a central POCT data management system fully integrated into the EMR (**Fig. 4**). Several companies are currently developing such a system.

Recent legislation to expand the use of EMRs[3] in place of paper files will emphasize the need for integration, as more clinicians, and soon, patients themselves, turn to the

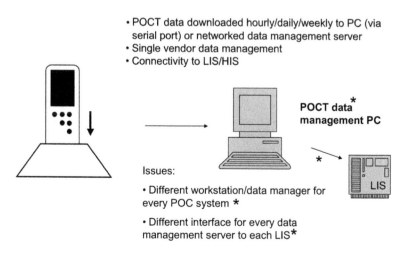

- POCT data downloaded hourly/daily/weekly to PC (via serial port) or networked data management server
- Single vendor data management
- Connectivity to LIS/HIS

POCT data*
management PC

Issues:

- Different workstation/data manager for every POC system *

- Different interface for every data management server to each LIS*

LIS

Fig. 2. Evolution of POCT connectivity, second generation. PC, personal computer; POC, point of care.

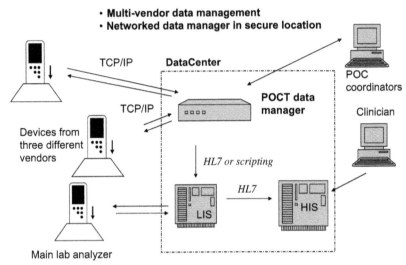

Fig. 3. Evolution of POCT connectivity, third generation. POC, point of care; TCP/IP, Transmission Control Protocol/Internet Protocol.

EMR as a single access point for laboratory results, whether for testing performed in the central laboratory or POCT performed at the patient's bedside. The EMR is rapidly becoming a comprehensive system, aggregating information from various clinical information systems, such as in anatomic pathology, laboratory medicine, radiology, and pharmacy. Cost-control efforts in health care reform are projected based on savings from EMRs and a new national health information technology infrastructure.[3–6] Incentives for coordination across the health care system using these electronic data systems will likely take on increasing importance in private and public payment schema. Health information exchange of all diagnostic data, whether

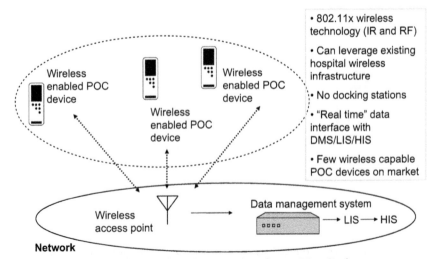

Fig. 4. Wireless POCT model. IR, infrared; POC, point of care; RF, radio frequency.

gathered in the central laboratory or near the patient, will play a key role in such inter-disciplinary management models, both within single institutions and across institutions. Thus, the problem of ensuring data connectivity will only become more important.

Current informatics-related problems in POCT include data communication, data generation, and data management. In the remainder of this article, we will review the structure of digital data and laboratory computer networks, discuss the importance of standards, and address ongoing efforts in POCT informatics regarding data communication, data generation, and data management.

DIGITAL DATA AND LABORATORY COMPUTER NETWORKS

To understand how data collected from a POCT device can be sent to a larger information system, such as the LIS, and eventually, the EMR, it is important to understand the nature of this data.[7] A typical pathology department will conduct more than a million laboratory tests a year in the central laboratory. In addition to the laboratory result, each test is associated with a patient, ordering clinician, the date and time testing was performed, and relevant quality control data and reference ranges, among other information. All data stored in computers is in binary code as a sequence of two numbers, 0 and 1. Binary code can be used to represent both numerical and textual data in the following ways.

The basic unit of digital storage is the *bit*, which is abbreviated from *binary digit* and can be represented by 0 or 1. A collection of eight bits is called a *byte*, and since each bit can hold one of two values, a byte can have 2^8 or 256 possible states. One byte, therefore, can represent any integer number from 0 to 255. Two bytes can identify integers between 0 and 65,535. Continuing in this logic, increasing aggregates of bytes can improve precision infinitely, while adding information, such as the positive or negative sign of the number.

Character data, or text, can be stored by representing each letter, symbol, or character as a coded number, which is then standardized for all fonts. The two most common codes for character data include the American Standard Code for Information Exchange (ASCII) and the Unicode Character Set. A set of numeric codes for a collection of letters (or symbols) will form a "string" in making up a word.

In the central laboratory, computer networks transfer data from a testing device to the LIS to report results and, in bidirectional manner, from the LIS to the device for ordering tests.[8] A computer network can be loosely defined as two devices sharing data over a medium, such as a cable wire (ie, copper, coaxial, fiber optic) or electromagnetic waves (ie, wireless). As reviewed above, all digital data is stored as 0's and 1's. On a wire, a series of 0's and 1's can be represented by a sequence of "high" and "low" voltages, respectively, transmitted over time. Signal quality relates to how closely together individual bits of data can be packed in time without degradation in the wire due to surrounding electrical interference. This depends on both the type of wire used as well as the distance over which the wire travels. The "bandwidth" of the network is also another way to think about signal quality, and refers to the amount of data that can be sent over time without signal degradation. Rates vary widely from 56 kilobits per second for dial-up modems to 100 megabits per second over Ethernet cables.[9]

The most common wireless networking standard is known as Wireless Fidelity, or "WiFi" or IEEE 802.11. In the United States, WiFi uses the 2.4-GHz frequency band, which is employed by many cordless telephones to transmit data via radio waves. The signal can pass through walls, ceilings, and floors, and this type of network is convenient for mobile users. However, wireless signals can be subject to interference, as well as easy access to data unless encrypted; achieving security for confidential patient information is an important consideration.

Central laboratory systems most often function in a secure wired network environment in the hospital, also known as a local area network (LAN). LIS network models include mainframe, client-server, and thin-client architectures.[8] The mainframe model uses a single computer to store data and perform software functions; users connect to the mainframe over the network via "dumb" terminals, which function solely as data-input and data-output devices. A client-server disperses the functions of the single computer in the mainframe model over several networked computers ("servers"). "Clients" are analogs to "dumb" terminals, and may be classified as "thick," "thin," or "hybrid," depending on how much of the data processing occurs on the client side versus the server. Thin clients depend on servers for the bulk of processing activities. Advantages to thin-client network architectures are that updates to software and hardware are easier to perform with centralized servers, and bandwidth requirements for networks may be less because there is less transfer of large files.

In contrast to central laboratories located in a defined space, the geographically dispersed nature of POCT presents a challenge to traditional hospital networks. The mobility of POCT users, who may or may not remember to regularly dock testing devices to a data management system to send results to the LIS, make wireless networks preferred. Devices may be programmed to automatically transmit and update information wirelessly to the data management system, no matter where the user is. Most likely, a combination of wireless and wired mediums will meet the needs of decentralized POCT. If segments of the communication from off-site testing areas occur over public networks, such as the Internet, it will also be critical to use secure methods, such as virtual private networks.

THE IMPORTANCE OF STANDARDS

Standards for data are pervasive in the modern world and help to transform data into useable information and, ultimately, knowledge. Previously mentioned examples of standards include ASCII and IEEE 802.11. When compliance is universal, standards are incredibly useful for data interpretation and transfer. Unfortunately, adherence to many standards is strictly voluntary and not always closely followed, particularly in health care.[10] Misinterpretation of data due to lack of adherence to a single standard can be disastrous. A famous example of this was the crash of the Mars Climate Orbiter on September 23, 1999, when metric units of measurement were given as input, but interpreted in the software as English units.[11]

In health care, poor standard implementation is fundamentally related to a number of current problems, including lack of interoperability of clinical information systems and inadequate data structuring.[10] Increasing recognition of the hazards of noncompliance or undercompliance to standards has led to bans on certain abbreviations in medical notes and prescriptions due to medication errors that occurred with nonstandard interpretations.[12] The US Institute of Medicine has recently advocated for standards that codify diagnostic data to reduce medical errors.[13]

Standards are particularly critical in laboratory testing. Laboratory data are highly structured in that a set of numbers for quality-control testing needs to be treated differently from those for a reference range, and to be interpreted separately from the results of testing. Therefore, when data are shared between two electronic devices, there must also be a way to embed meaning in the data so that the various data elements are not confused with one another. This is commonly performed in the central laboratory using Health Level 7 (HL7), a standard messaging protocol that provides identifiers to data elements.

HL7 is a message standard widely used in the health care environment (www.HL7. org). Many current LISs use version 2.x, which identifies data by their positions in a string of characters. The meaning of these positions is defined by the HL7 standard. Start and stop markers for positions are also defined by special characters called *delimiters*, such as a vertical bar ("|") or the caret ("^"). Thus, even if a data field were to be blank, delimiters would still need to be included so that subsequent fields are interpreted appropriately.

Extensible Markup Language (XML) is the basis for HL7 version 3.0, and is a general-purpose meta-language created by the World Wide Web Consortium (W3C) for the purpose of data exchange.[14] XML has yet to be implemented in many LISs, but promises to provide greater flexibility in data sharing. XML consists of a set of user-defined tags represented within angle-brackets ("< >") that annotate the data. For example, the XML tag <state> can be defined in a separate metadocument explaining the data element as consisting of two uppercase characters used to describe one of the 50 states in the United States. Tags can be used in the following manner to denote the start and end of the relevant data element in a patient file:

<state>MA</state>

The separate metadocument defining the tags can then be matched to another set of user-defined tags in a different clinical information system; this may allow for sharing of data across health care institutions. Such tags may even be used in diagnostic narrative reports, such as in anatomic pathology or radiology reports, to provide structure for search functions.

Similar to standards for data interpretation (ie, HL7), shared network protocols are also key for data communication. For example, without a shared network protocol, two data packets sent simultaneously from opposite ends of a wired network may collide and result in transmission errors. Ethernet, a network protocol commonly used in hospital networks, is based on a "contention" logic called *carrier-sense/ multiple access—collision detection* or *CSMA/CD*.[15] In this protocol, when a device is about to transmit its data packet, it first "listens" to the network to see if there is another message being communicated. If so, it waits for that message to be sent before it sends its own packet of data. If a collision occurs, both "speakers" stop transmitting and go into a random "wait period" before trying again. Using this protocol, 70% to 80% of the theoretical bandwidth based on the hardware (ie, cable, wireless signal) can be achieved.

POC CONNECTIVITY STANDARD

Historically, a well-described barrier to POCT integration with the central LIS and/or HIS was the lack of a standard for universal connectivity.[16] A 1998 survey by the American Association for Clinical Chemistry Point-of-Care Testing Division revealed that "connectivity" and "data management" were two aspects of POCT that were of greatest concern to staff. A follow-up survey of more than 500 United States hospitals by Enterprise Corporation for the American Association of Clinical Chemistry revealed that 67% of POCT data never reached the LIS, and only 15% of POCT data was sent to the LIS electronically.[17] Nonpublished surveys suggest that less than 10% of hospitals send POCT data to the EMR.[18]

Typically, many hospitals employ POCT instruments from multiple vendors, including manually performed, visually read tests, as shown in **Box 1**. Multivendor data

---

Box 1
POCTs performed at the Massachusetts General Hospital

Instrumented tests

    Bedside glucose testing

    Urinalysis (Clinitek 50 status)

    Hemocue hemoglobin

    Blood gases, electrolytes, lactate

    Activated clotting time

    Co-oximetry

    Cardiac markers

    Urine drugs of abuse

    D-dimer

    Creatinine

Manually performed visually read tests

    Fecal occult blood

    Urine pregnancy testing

    Rapid strep A

    Rapid influenza A/B

    Rapid respiratory syncytial virus

    Nitrazine paper test

    Gram stain

    Potassium hydroxide preparation

    Joint crystal examination

---

connectivity across a hospital campus has proved very challenging, despite availability of open architecture enterprise POCT data management software from several vendors. Currently, there is no satisfactory solution for managing manual POCTs, such as fecal occult blood testing or urinalysis, unless these tests can be converted to an instrument-read device. These tests still require error-prone hand-written records or manual data entry into the POCT data management system. For all of these reasons, achieving the goal of true POCT connectivity remains very much a work in progress.

Vendor-neutral enterprise POCT data management systems require significant capital investment, many being expensive to install and incurring ongoing costs associated with software licensing, maintenance, and upgrades. Alternatively, systems supplied by device manufacturers may be free (or low cost), but may not be vendor-neutral or may only be able to interface to a limited number of alternative devices. Of course, the true cost of these vendor-supplied systems is ultimately included in the price for the devices, the consumables, or both.

Another expensive option is to interface each POCT device directly to the LIS. This type of interface typically costs from $5000 to $10,000. In situations where the test volume is small, the incremental cost per test can be prohibitive. For example, a device that performs 25 tests per day over a 5-year lifespan of the instrument, assuming an interface cost of $7,500, would incur an interface cost per test of approximately

16 cents. On the other hand, for a device performing only one test per day, the interface cost per test would be $4.11. This latter number would be cost-prohibitive in most situations. Regardless of the solution used, achieving POCT connectivity is very expensive across a large hospital campus. In low-volume settings, the cost of connectivity may be unacceptable.

In early 2000, the Connectivity Industry Consortium (CIC) was created by a group of vendors, hospitals, and POCT experts to develop a POCT connectivity standard that would reduce the burden of integrating results from diagnostic devices from different vendors. The goals of the CIC were to address issues of bidirectional communication, standardized "plug-and-play" device connections, software interoperability, security, and regulatory compliance, and to use existing standards and infrastructure whenever possible.[19] The resulting specifications were subsequently approved in 2001 by the National Committee for Clinical Laboratory Standards (NCCLS, now named Clinical and Laboratory Standards Institute or CLSI; www.clsi.org) as the POCT1-A standard, with a recently updated second edition in 2006 as POCT1-A2.[20]

The POCT1-A standard describes two interfaces involving POCT devices and information systems, namely the *device interface* and the *observation reporting interface*.[21] The device interface is involved in the communication between devices and their related data management systems, such as docking stations. The observation reporting interface guides the information exchange between data managers and a central information system, such as the LIS or a clinical data repository, from which results may be viewed and into which data may be stored.

The device interface consists of two parts: (1) a common messaging schema for the dialog between the device and its data manager (device messaging layer specification [DMS]) and (2) a technical protocol for reliable communication of the data (device and access point specification [DAP]). At a minimum for all devices, DMS messages must include the device status and observations (eg, patient results, quality control results). Additional optional message types include device events (eg, errors, uncertified operators), list updates (eg, new operator, new patient), and directives for lock-outs or vendor-specific messages. All messages are to be encoded in XML, which now forms the basis for version 3.0 of HL7, which many laboratory systems have yet to convert to.

The DAP describes physical interfaces and protocols used to connect to POCT devices. Tiny Transport protocol (TinyTP) was chosen as a low-cost widely available solution that could be run over infrared signals or cables, both having strongly established prior standards.

The observation reporting interface is designed to address the specific workflow needs around the ordering process for POCT devices. Using HL7-based messages currently used in the central laboratory for instrument communication, this interface handles the search and matching of orders to POCT results and, in many cases, the generation of orders when no preexisting orders can be found.

All standards must be updated periodically. Existing standards groups are involved in maintaining and updating POCT1-A.[22] The Institute for Electrical and Electronics Engineers (IEEE, www.ieee.org) maintains specifications related to the physical connection and protocols between instruments and data managers. HL7 manages the standards for messaging communications between data managers and the LIS. The recent approved second edition; POCT1-A2; now has an expanded section related to radio frequency (RF) networking.

It is anticipated that incorporation of the POCT1-A2 standard in future POCT devices will allow for easier interoperability with the LIS and HIS for results and orders.

POCT DATA GENERATION AND MANAGEMENT

Developments in POCT informatics have the potential to affect problems related to patient safety and quality control by generating or managing data previously eliminated or ignored in the POCT workflow. Reduced turnaround time in POCT to provide "just-in-time" data has been achieved through the elimination of a number of steps commonly performed for testing in the central laboratory, such as order-entry and quality control documentation.

The order-entry step is important in providing identifying information for the patient, ordering physician, and the test to be performed, along with other data (eg, relevant clinical history, date and time of specimen collection). Recording the order is also essential for billing purposes, and billing for POCT has been unsuccessful in many institutions because of lack of reliable documentation practices for order entry.[18]

POCT devices must have the operator provide identifying information while balancing the user's demand for convenience and rapid results. Various informatics strategies have been proposed to address this issue.[23] Currently available technologies, such as bar codes on operator identification badges and patient wristbands, can accurately and efficiently capture identifying information, and may form part of the solution. Through the use of "intelligent" messages and/or "lock-outs," user interfaces can also be carefully designed for correction of preanalytic errors. This type of guidance may help avoid data-input errors, such as errors that indicate a test was performed on one patient, when it was actually performed on another.

Equally problematic have been failures to properly document for quality controls and to collect data required to maintain regulatory compliance. These failures stem in part from complex and, in some cases, unique regulatory requirements for POCT.[18] Inadequate validation and quality assurance measures for test results may lead to compromises in patient safety and issues of medical-legal liability. Problems with POCT have been frequently reported in the past, with self-monitoring glucose devices scoring the highest number of complaints filed with the Food and Drug Administration out of all medical devices in the 1990s.[24]

For quality assurance purposes, technical conditions present at the time of testing, including reagent lot numbers, calibrator expiration dates, reference ranges, quality control results, and test validation records, must be recorded and archived with the analytic results. Messages and lock-outs can also be used to manage compliance with quality control testing. An additional requirement for quality control purposes is a bidirectional communication interface between the testing device and the LIS. Such an interface can send data from the LIS to inform the testing device of changes in reagent lot numbers, new quality control ranges, patient registration data, and the list of users authorized to perform testing, among other important information. A universal bidirectional interface between POCT devices and the LIS via a data management system is a key component of the recent POCT1-A connectivity standard, discussed previously.

ONGOING AND FUTURE POCT INFORMATICS NEEDS

The full benefits from the POCT1-A standard are yet to be seen with widespread adoption of standard-compliant devices. The integration of data from POCT devices with those of other clinical information systems holds the promise of expanding the role of the laboratory in disease management and clinical decision support. Still, issues remain regarding current POCT devices and their data management systems, as well as regarding the broader hospital information technology environment.[25]

Enterprise POCT data management systems are now available from several companies and include both open-architecture and closed-architecture systems. Examples of open-architecture vendor-neutral systems include the Remote Automated Laboratory System (RALS) and Telcor, which are sold as software systems independent of purchases of testing devices or reagents. Closed-architecture systems supplied by a device manufacturer as part of the purchase of their testing products include Rapidlink (Siemens), Medisense Precision Net (Abbott Diagnostics), and Gem Web (Instrumentation Laboratories). Some manufacturer-supplied systems are capable of interfacing to products supplied by other instrument vendors. Many hospitals have purchased dedicated POCT data management systems to manage information from multiple devices from different manufacturers. However, these systems have not achieved the goal of true plug-and-play connectivity, even though most of these POCT data management systems have preconfigured off-the-shelf interfaces for many different POCT devices.

A significant part of the problem is the information technology environment in which these POCT systems must operate. It is not simply sufficient to connect the point-of-care device to the data management system. When the POCT system is embedded into an existing hospital network, it is necessary to enable data to flow from multiple hospital information systems, such as the billing system, the hospital admissions/discharge/transfer system, the LIS, and the hospital patient care information system. Major challenges can occur when data must flow seamlessly across the entire hospital network. As a result, getting a new device connected to the network may prove extremely challenging.

Furthermore, even when the data can finally be made to flow through the network, other problems may arise. For example, some instruments record testing data in real time but only transmit the results when the device is connected to a docking station. The LIS may not be capable of recognizing these tests as having been ordered and performed in the past. The result is that the LIS creates an order and posts a result reflecting the time that docking occurred, thereby assigning a wrong date or time to the test result. Test results that may be hours or several days old suddenly appear as a bolus in the EMR, creating confusion for clinicians.

In other situations, the hospital information technology infrastructure may be deficient. For example, when we attempted to implement POCT for blood gases and electrolytes in our operating rooms, we ran into several major problems. First, the data management server used by one manufacturer did not meet the standards set by our information technology department. The information technology group declined to support the server. We could have used an off-site server "farm" for this purpose, but the cost was excessive. We chose an alternate vendor for our POCT devices, only to discover that the operating rooms did not have the proper wiring infrastructure to support the data management system. The cost to retrofit the operating rooms approached $100,000 and delayed the project by 6 months.

These examples illustrate a key problem in POCT data management. Highly functional POCT information technology solutions developed by vendors cannot anticipate all of the myriad issues that can arise when these systems are installed in an existing information technology environment. The issues include both problems with existing software in the hospital and with the hospital's hardware infrastructure.

A large number of different health care information systems exist across the country. Many of these are hybrids of different systems supplied by various software vendors to create an information technology network. Some of the systems are home grown or highly modified commercial systems. Given this information technology environment, achieving POCT connectivity will continue to be a major challenge.

One promising solution to the dilemma of POCT connectivity is wireless communication. In concept, this technology would eliminate many of the barriers to achieving true real-time POCT data connectivity. There will, of course, be challenges that need to be overcome, not least of which is that many devices are not yet wireless-enabled, and many hospital sites are not yet equipped to handle wireless data communication. A number of companies are working on wireless POCT data connectivity solutions. Several of these companies supply POC devices for bedside glucose testing. As in the past, the connectivity needs associated with bedside glucose testing may well be the driver of next-generation connectivity leading the field of POCT into the future of wireless connectivity.

SUMMARY

Managing patient test data and documenting regulatory compliance for tests performed at the point of care has traditionally been a significant problem. In many situations, manual recordkeeping has proven entirely inadequate to maintain the integrity of the patient medical record or to provide an audit trail for quality assurance activities. Starting in the 1990s, a number of companies began to develop and market point-of-care data management systems. Over time, these data management systems have become increasingly sophisticated. It is now possible to interface multiple point-of-care devices from different manufacturers to a central data manager that is bidirectionally interfaced to the laboratory and hospital information systems. Despite these advances, many challenges remain. True real-time POC "connectivity" across an entire institution has yet to be achieved, and there is still no satisfactory solution for manually performed visually read tests, some of which are commonly performed at the point of care. In the future, wireless POC connectivity solutions hold great promise, but these technologies are yet to be fully developed.

REFERENCES

1. Nichols JH. Point-of-care testing: performance improvement and evidence-based outcomes. New York: Marcel Dekker; 2003.
2. Halpern NA. Point of care diagnostics and networks. Crit Care Clin 2000;16(4): 623–39.
3. Blumenthal D. Stimulating the adoption of health information technology. N Engl J Med 2009;360(15):1477–9.
4. Blumenthal D, Glaser J. Information technology comes to medicine. N Engl J Med 2007;356(24):2527–34.
5. Mongan J, Ferris T, Lee T. Options for slowing the growth of health care costs. N Engl J Med 2008;358(14):1509–14.
6. Hillestad R, Bigelow J, Bower A, et al. Can electronic medical record systems transform health care? Potential health benefits, savings, and costs. Health Aff 2005;24(5):1103–17.
7. Sinard JH. Chapter 2: desktop computers: hardware, chapter 3: desktop computers: software. In: Practical pathology informatics: demystifying informatics for the practicing anatomic pathologist. New York, NY: Springer Science+Business Media, Inc.; 2006. p. 21–3, 72–3.
8. Pantanowitz L, Henricks WH, Beckwith BA. Medical laboratory informatics. Clin Lab Med 2007;27(4):823–43, vii.
9. Smith MB. Introduction to telepathology. In: Cowan DF, editor. Informatics for the clinical laboratory: a practical guide for the pathologist. New York, NY: Springer; 2005. p. 268–86.

10. Berman JJ. Chapter 4: standards for biomedical data. In: Biomedical informatics. Sudbury (MA): Jones and Bartlett; 2007. p. 61–91.
11. Mars climate orbiter mishap investigation board phase I report. November 10, 1999. Available at: ftp://ftp.hq.nasa.gov/pub/pao/reports/1999/MCO_report.pdf.
12. Booker DL, Berman JJ. Dangerous abbreviations. Hum Pathol 2004;35(5): 529–31.
13. Aspden P. Institute of Medicine (U.S.). Committee on data standards for patient safety. Patient safety: achieving a new standard for care. Washington (DC): National Academies Press; 2004.
14. Berman JJ. Pathology data integration with eXtensible Markup Language. Hum Pathol 2005;36(2):139–45.
15. Sinard JH. Chapter 4: networking and the Internet. In: Practical pathology informatics: demystifying informatics for the practicing anatomic pathologist. New York, NY: Springer Science+Business Media, Inc.; 2006. p. 95–8.
16. Jones R, St. John A. Informatics in point-of-care testing. In: Price CP, St. John A, Hicks JM, editors. Point-of-care testing. 2nd edition. Washington (DC): AACC Press; 2004. p. 197–208.
17. Stephens EJ. Developing open standards for point-of-care connectivity. IVD Technology: for In vitro Diagnostics Development & Manufacturing 1999;10: 22–5.
18. Blick K. The essential role of information management in point-of-care/critical care testing. Clin Chim Acta 2001;307(1–2):159–68.
19. Nichols JH. The connectivity industry consortium standard. Point of Care 2002; 1(2):109–10.
20. Clinical and Laboratory Standards Institute (CLSI). Point-of-Care Connectivity; Approved Standard. 2nd edition. CLSI document POCT1-A2 (ISBN 1-56238-616-6). Wayne (PA): Clinical and Laboratory Standards Institute; 2006. p. 1–306.
21. Perry J, Anders B, Boecker D. Point-of-care testing integration and connectivity. In: Kost GJ, editor. Principles & practice of point-of-care testing. Philadelphia: Lippincott Williams & Wilkins; 2002. p. 507–15.
22. Uleski RC. Advances in connectivity standards for point of care testing. Point of Care 2002;1(2):117–8.
23. Jones JB. Chapter 3: information management of point-of-care testing: strategies for improving outcomes. In: Nichols JH, editor. Point-of-care testing: performance improvement and evidence-based outcomes. New York: Marcel Dekker; 2003. p. 59–99.
24. Greyson J. Quality control in patient self-monitoring of blood glucose. Diabetes Care 1993;16(9):1306–8.
25. Safely implementing health information and converging technologies. Jt Comm Perspect 2009;29(1):10–3.

Regulatory Compliance for Point-of-Care Testing: 2009 United States Perspective

Sharon S. Ehrmeyer, PhD, MT(ASCP)[a],*, Ronald H. Laessig, PhD[b]

KEYWORDS

- Clinical Laboratory Improvement Amendments
- Point-of-care testing compliance • Regulatory compliance
- Testing requirements • Professional accreditation

All clinical laboratory testing in the United States, regardless of where performed, is regulated by the Clinical Laboratory Improvement Amendments of 1988 (CLIA'88 or CLIA) and overseen by the Centers for Medicare and Medicaid Services (CMS).[1] The current CLIA regulatory requirements are specified in the January 24, 2003, "Final Rule."[2] A companion document, *Survey Procedures and Interpretive Guidelines for Laboratories and Laboratory Services in the State Operations Manual* (published January 2004) further clarifies each requirement and identifies what activities CMS inspectors expect test sites to do to meet these requirements.[3]

CLIA profoundly changed the prevailing United States regulatory philosophy by imposing uniform requirements for all clinical laboratory testing regardless of where tests are performed. This "site-neutral" approach means that for any particular test (eg, a cardiac marker, blood glucose, or a urine dipstick), whether it is performed at a large reference laboratory, a major clinic, a local hospital, a small physician office laboratory, or at the patient's bedside, is subject to the same regulations. The clear intent of the "site-neutral" CLIA regulations is to ensure that all clinical laboratory testing meets a minimum standard of quality. Conceptually, all patients are entitled to quality laboratory results, regardless of where, when, or who performs the tests.

CLIA specifies minimum testing requirements for every site examining "materials derived from the human body for the purpose of providing information for the diagnosis, prevention, or treatment of any disease..."[2] While CLIA sets the minimum requirements and CMS inspects sites for compliance, voluntary accreditation through

[a] Clinical Laboratory Science/Medical Technology Program, Department of Pathology and Laboratory Medicine, University of Wisconsin School of Medicine and Public Health, Madison, WI 53706, USA
[b] Department of Population Health Sciences, Wisconsin State Laboratory of Hygiene, University of Wisconsin School of Medicine and Public Health, Madison, WI 53706, USA
* Corresponding author.
E-mail address: ehrmeyer@wisc.edu (S.S. Ehrmeyer).

Clin Lab Med 29 (2009) 463–478
doi:10.1016/j.cll.2009.06.012
0272-2712/09/$ – see front matter © 2009 Elsevier Inc. All rights reserved.

labmed.theclinics.com

professional organizations "deemed" by CMS to have equivalent or more stringent requirements than those specified in the CLIA is an alternative for point-of-care testing (POCT) sites. POCT sites in hospitals usually meet the CLIA requirements by being accredited and inspected by one of these professional organizations, primarily the Joint Commission, the Laboratory Accreditation Program of the College of American Pathologists (LAP-CAP), or Cola (formerly known as the Commission on Office Laboratory Accreditation).[4–6] Professional organizations charge a fee for inspection, assessment, and accreditation. When POCT sites meet the accrediting agency's requirements, as assessed through inspection every 2 years, the test site also meets the CLIA requirements. The CMS, however, has the right, for quality-assurance purposes, to reinspect up to 5% of testing sites accredited by CMS-deemed organizations. While each organization has a slightly different approach to conducting the inspection, the accreditation standards must be fully compliant with the CLIA regulations. Test sites have the option of selecting the accrediting organization. However, POCT sites must be cognizant of the basic CLIA requirements as well as all applicable professional accreditation standards, guidelines, or checklists.

CLINICAL LABORATORY IMPROVEMENT AMENDMENTS OF 1988 CERTIFICATES

The first requirement for any POCT site is to perform testing under an appropriate and current CLIA certificate.[7] Some sites mistakenly think that no CLIA certificate is necessary when patients are not charged for the testing. This is not true. The holder of the CLIA certificate for a POCT site within a hospital typically fits into one of two broad scenarios: (1) the central laboratory holds a single CLIA certificate that covers all institutional testing, including POCT, or (2) POCT sites within the institution have their own, separate CLIA certificates. There is no one right way; the choice most often depends on policy, administrative concerns, and cost. Free-standing POCT sites, such as physician office laboratories, including those in multiphysician practices (clinics), must have their own CLIA certificates. CLIA certificates are based in part on the complexity of the methods. Complexity is determined by the technical difficulty and the knowledge, skills, and experience necessary to perform the testing. Because of personnel and quality requirements, usually only waived or moderate-complexity methods are used at the point of care. However, if a POCT site develops its own test procedure or chooses to modify an existing procedure approved by the Food and Drug Administration (FDA)—such as deviating from the manufacturer's directions—the method automatically falls into the high-complexity category and is subject to CLIA's most stringent requirements. The cost of CLIA certificates for independent test sites is determined by a CMS fee schedule, which is set according to test volume, specialty/subspecialty of testing, and test-complexity level.[8]

The FDA places each test method into one of three categories: waived, moderate complexity, and high complexity. However, in the 2003 regulations, the CMS combined many requirements relating to moderate- and high-complexity test methods and sometimes refers to these two categories as *nonwaived*. Primarily because of personnel and method-validation requirements, the waived category has the least stringent testing requirements while the high-complexity level has the most stringent. Moderate complexity includes the subcategory of provider-performed microscopy procedures (PPMP), which is designated specifically for physician and midlevel practitioner testing as part of their professional practice of medicine.[9] The limited test menu for this category consists of wet mount preparations for the presence or absence of bacteria, fungi, parasites, and human cellular elements; potassium hydroxide preparations; pinworm examinations; fern tests; postcoital direct qualitative examinations of vaginal or cervical mucous; urine sediment examinations; nasal smears for granulocytes; fecal leukocyte examinations; and qualitative semen analysis. The instrument for performing PPMP tests is the microscope. Practitioners testing under a CLIA-PPMP certificate can do these procedures as well as waived tests, but no others. To do moderate- or high-complexity tests, the test site must have an appropriate "registration" certificate and meet specific quality, personnel, and other requirements.

POCT sites wanting their own certificate need to apply by filling out the CMS 116 form available on the CMS Web site.[10] Test sites specify one of the following categories:

Waiver: a certificate that permits a site to perform only those tests methods identified as waived

PPMP: a certificate that permits only physicians, midlevel practitioners, or dentists to perform any of the nine PPMP procedures on specimens collected during a physical examination as well as all of the waived tests

Registration: a certificate issued to enable test sites to conduct waived, moderate-complexity, and/or high-complexity test methodologies

Once the site is judged through inspection to be "CLIA compliant," a renewable certificate of compliance is issued. POCT sites specifically seeking accreditation by a CMS-deemed professional organization are issued a certificate of accreditation upon passing inspection.[7] As of 2008, approximately 207,000 CLIA certificates had been issued.[11] Eight percent of the testing sites are accredited and inspected by professional accrediting agencies. The central laboratory and POCT sites within the same institution *may* be accredited by different organizations. CMS also recognizes two "CLIA-exempt" states, Washington and New York, as having requirements at least equivalent to those of the CLIA; test sites within these states must meet the specific state's requirements. All other states inspect sites on behalf of CMS using the 2003 CLIA regulations and 2004 *State Operations Manual* guidelines; they may also impose additional criteria (eg, California's personnel requirements).

Regulatory Guidelines

The CLIA law (Public Law, 1988) specifies that testing requirements are to be based on complexity of the test method performed.[1] The US Congress specifically excluded a limited number of test procedures and "waived" CMS regulatory oversight if certain requirements are met. CLIA originally defined *waived* as "tests cleared by the Food and Drug Administration (FDA) for home use" (ie, tests that patients can purchase over the counter) and "tests using such simple and accurate methodologies that the likelihood of erroneous results is negligible."[2] In 1992, when the CLIA requirements were first published in the *Federal Register,* only eight analytes were waived: dipstick/tablet reagent urinalysis (visually read), fecal occult blood, visual urine pregnancy and ovulation tests, nonautomated erythrocyte sedimentation rate, blood glucose by monitoring devices cleared by the FDA for home use, hemoglobin by copper sulfate, and spun hematocrit. In 1993, hemoglobin—analyzed by single analyte instruments with direct measurement and readout—was added. In 1997, the US Congress provided a mechanism for manufacturers to apply for waiver status. The FDA recently updated this mechanism.[12] The waived list continues to grow and currently includes more than 100 analytes measured by multiple specific methods or "kits." The official list of all commercial, waived test methods is available on the CMS Web site and from the labeling information provided by reagent and instrument manufacturers.[13]

Waived testing under Clinical Laboratory Improvement Amendments of 1988
For POCT sites performing only waived testing and not seeking accreditation from a professional organization, CLIA has no specific personnel, quality control, or quality assessment requirements other than to follow the manufacturers' directions (**Table 1**). For some methods, however, manufacturers have specific requirements, such as the periodic analysis of quality-control materials. The CMS inspectors responsible for determining how well POCT sites adhere to CLIA regulations will not inspect waived testing sites unless a specific complaint has been lodged or fraudulent activities are suspected.

Moderate-complexity testing under Clinical Laboratory Improvement Amendments of 1988
Of the test methods currently being marketed, more than half are classified by the FDA as moderate complexity. POCT sites performing any moderate-complexity test must meet regulatory requirements set out in the following sections (**Table 2**).

Personnel (Clinical Laboratory Improvement Amendments of 1988 sections [2003 Federal Register] §493.1403–25) For POCT sites holding their own CLIA certificates and performing moderately complex testing, individuals with the proper qualifications must be identified for the positions of director, technical consultant, clinical consultant, and testing personnel. Some point-of-care sites with their own certificate may have one individual fill several personnel positions. Alternatively, when POCT falls under the central laboratory's certificate, typically only the testing personnel requirements need to be addressed at point of care because the required oversight is from the central laboratory. The director, as listed on the CLIA certificate, can be a physician; someone with a bachelor's degree in medical technology/clinical laboratory science; or someone with a degree in chemical, physical, or biologic science and 2 years of laboratory training/experience and 2 years of laboratory supervisory experience. The director is responsible for all aspects of POCT operation and administration. Although he or she may delegate the duties to qualified individuals, the director is ultimately responsible for ensuring that all duties are properly performed. The POCT site also must have one or more individuals qualified by education and either training or experience to provide technical consultation for each of the specialties and subspecialties of service in which the point of care performs moderate-complexity test procedures. The technical consultant establishes the quality standards for the POCT site. These include standards related to selecting and monitoring methods/instrumentation and evaluating and documenting the competency of the personnel. A technical consultant can be, for example, a clinician or an individual possessing a bachelor's degree in chemical, physical, biologic, or medical technology/clinical laboratory science and 1 year of laboratory training or experience in the designated specialty of responsibility. The clinical consultant must be a clinician or have a doctorate in chemical, physical, biologic, or medical technology/clinical laboratory science. This person serves as the liaison between the POCT site and its customers. This individual must be qualified to consult with clinicians and patients and give opinions concerning the diagnosis, treatment, and management of patient care. The testing personnel are responsible for specimen processing, test performance, and reporting test results. Minimum requirements for testing personnel include a high school education or equivalent plus appropriate, director-approved training and ongoing (at least yearly) competency assessment. In some POCT situations, an individual, such as a physician directing a physician office laboratory, depending on qualifications, may fill multiple positions.

Procedure manual (Clinical Laboratory Improvement Amendments of 1988 sections [2003 Federal Register] §493.1251) The number one CLIA deficiency cited by inspectors is failure to follow manufacturers' directions. Consequently, complete "standard operating procedures" are essential. In written or in electronic form, they must be available to all testing personnel for all tests performed. The necessary elements, as appropriate for the method, include written policies and procedures for patient preparation; specimen collection, labeling, preservation, transportation, referral, and rejection criteria; directions for step-by-step performance of the procedure; instrument calibration and calibration verification; reportable range; quality control and corrective actions; limitations of the methodology; reference intervals; critical values; literature references; reporting of patient results; and course of action when a test system becomes inoperable. Manufacturers' product inserts or operator manuals may be used to substantially meet this requirement. However, additional information specific to the POCT site must be included. Initially, the procedures must be approved, signed, and dated by the POCT site director. Any changes to the procedures or changes in directorship require reapproval by the current director. The Clinical and Laboratory Standards Institute (CLSI) document, *The CLSI Procedure Manual Toolkit: Improving Procedure Writing in the Clinical Laboratory (GPO2-A5-C)*, describes the framework for developing procedures and communicating and organizing information.[14]

Control procedures (Clinical Laboratory Improvement Amendments of 1988 sections [2003 Federal Register] §493.1256) CLIA section §493.1256 begins with the statement: "For each test system, the laboratory is responsible for having control procedures that monitor the accuracy and precision of the complete analytical process." According to this section, the test's control procedures must (1) detect immediate errors that occur due to test system failure, adverse environmental conditions, and operator performance, and (2) monitor, over time, the accuracy and precision of the test procedure that may be influenced by changes in test system performance, environmental conditions, and variance in operator performance. For most quantitative and qualitative moderately complex tests performed at the point of care, the minimum requirement for full CLIA compliance is two levels of liquid quality control per 24 hours unless the manufacturer requires more. However, section §493.1256(d), which is new with the 2003 CLIA revisions, allows for an alternative quality-control procedure, provided it is approved by the CMS and provides equivalent quality testing as specified in "Appendix C" of the (2004) *State Operations Manual*. This equivalent-quality testing is now termed *equivalent quality control* or *EQC*. This section clearly was designed to address many of the instruments used at the point of care that incorporate built-in quality-assessment capabilities. Conceptually, EQC empowers manufacturers to design and integrate into their instruments or test systems automated quality-assessment protocols based on internal or process controls, which, independent of the operator, carry out quality-control and quality-assurance functions. Once a test site demonstrates, using one of the three EQC evaluation options identified in "Appendix C" of the 2004 *State Operations Manual*, that the manufacturer's approach is sufficiently robust for evaluation of instrument accuracy and precision, the test site's director can rely on the EQC approach and only run external, liquid controls every 7 days or 30 days, depending on the evaluation option selected. The evaluation options consist of running traditional, external quality control in parallel with the manufacturer's internal quality-control protocol for 10, 30, or 60 days and having the director review the comparative data.[3] If acceptable, the director signs off on the evaluation and allows the POCT site to use EQC instead of external controls for daily quality assessment.

Table 1
Comparison of waived testing requirements by deemed-accrediting organization

Requirement	CMS (CLIA)	Cola Accreditation	Joint Commission Accreditation	LAP-CAP Accreditation
CLIA certificate	Yes, based on complexity level of test performed	Same as for CLIA	Same as for CLIA	Same as for CLIA
General requirements for test methods	Follow manufacturers' directions	Same as for CLIA	Follow waived testing standards in current Laboratory Accreditation Standards	Follow applicable standards in current Laboratory General Checklist and Point-of-Care Testing Checklists
Quality control	Follow manufacturers' directions	Same as for CLIA	Follow manufacturers' directions; if not stated, define frequency of quality control; for instrument-based procedures, run at least 2 quality control levels each day of testing; document all quality-control results	Follow manufacturers' directions; review quality control daily and at least monthly by director or designee; document unacceptable internal quality control results unless instrument has "lock-out" to prevent release of patient data; verify quality control before reporting results; perform and document corrective action when quality control exceeds limits
Validation of manufacturer's "built-in" EQC approach	No	No	No	No

Mandated personnel training/competency assessment	No	No	Yes; documented training for each test authorized to perform and competency assessment after orientation to testing and annually thereafter	Yes; documented training for each test authorized to perform and competency assessment after orientation to testing and annually thereafter
Validation of method's performance specifications	No	No	No, unless required by manufacturer or organization	No, unless required by manufacturer or organization
Policies and procedures (standard operating procedures)	Testing personnel are expected to follow manufacturer's instructions	Same as for CLIA	Yes; must be current and complete and include specimen type, collection and handling, instrument maintenance and function checks, quality control, and any other institution-specific procedure associated with test performance; director approves before initial use and at least every 3 y and when changes are made	Yes; current and complete and should address preanalytical, analytical, and postanalytical considerations; at least annual review by director or designee
Test result records	No (good laboratory practice requires documentation in patient record)	Same as for CLIA	Yes; documented in the clinical record and quantitative results accompanied by reference interval	Yes; retained in permanent medical record and accompanied, when applicable, by reference intervals or interpretive ranges
Proficiency testing	No	No	No	Yes, if available; when not available, perform semiannual, alternative accuracy assessment
Inspection	No, unless complaint is received or fraud suspected	Yes; will check for adherence to manufacturer's directions	Yes; for compliance to the 5 waived testing standards	Yes; for compliance to the appropriate Laboratory General Checklist and Point-of-Care Testing Checklist items

Table 2
Moderate-complexity testing requirements by deemed-accrediting organization[a]

Requirement	CMS (CLIA)	Cola Accreditation	Joint Commission Accreditation	LAP-CAP Accreditation
General requirements for test methods	Follow manufacturer's directions; have policies and procedures in place for the preanalytical, analytical, and postanalytical phases of testing	Same as for CLIA	Same as for CLIA	Same as for CLIA
Procedure manual (standard operating procedures)	Written policies and procedures, as appropriate from patient preparation to reporting (§493.1251); approved by director initially and with any changes	Same as for CLIA	Same as for CLIA; approved by director initially and with any changes; reapproved annually	Same as for CLIA; approved by director initially and with any changes; reapproved annually
Quality control	Follow section §493.1256 for general requirements and §§493.1261, 1267, 1269, and 1254 for analyte-specific requirements: general requirement: 2 quality-control levels/test/d	Follow, as applicable, general quality-control section and test specialty requirements in current COLA Laboratory Accreditation Criteria manual	Follow, as applicable, general quality-control and test specialty standards in current Laboratory Accreditation Standards	Follow, as applicable, quality-control and test specialty standards in current Point-of Care Checklist

Accepts manufacturer's internal/procedural/on-board EQC approach to fulfill daily quality control requirements	Yes, once qualified by one of 3 EQC validation options (identified in 2004 State Operations Manual)	Yes; qualify approach by either a 10- or 30-d evaluation	Yes; qualify approach for routine chemistry or hematology with a 10- or 30-d evaluation	Yes; qualify approach with a 20-d evaluation study for devices with built-in liquid controls; for devices with electronic or process controls, follow protocol defined by director
Proficiency testing in a CMS-approved proficiency-testing program/accuracy assessment	Yes; follow, as appropriate §§493.801–865 for regulated analytes; when proficiency testing is not performed, then an accuracy assessment (§493.1236(c)) must be made at least every 6 mo	Essentially the same as for CLIA, but follow Cola standards	Essentially the same as for CLIA, but follow Joint Commission standards	For all analytes tested, when proficiency testing is available; when not available, assess accuracy at least every 6 mo
Personnel qualifications	Follow §§493.1403–1425	Same as for CLIA	Same as for CLIA	Same as for CLIA
Testing personnel training and on-going competency assessment	Yes; technical consultant (or director) is responsible for identifying (initial) training needs and ongoing competency assessments (§493.1403[7][8])	Same as for CLIA	Same as for CLIA	

(continued on next page)

Table 2
(continued)

Requirement	CMS (CLIA)	Cola Accreditation	Joint Commission Accreditation	LAP-CAP Accreditation
Initial method verification at start-up	Follow §493.1253 (accuracy, precision, reportable range, and approve acceptability of reportable range)	Same as for CLIA	Same as for CLIA	Same as for CLIA
Ongoing assessment of reportable range (every 6 mo)	Yes; §493.1255(b)(3) (accomplished through calibration verification)	Same as for CLIA	Same as for CLIA	Same as for CLIA (termed *analytical measurement range [AMR]*)
Quality assessment: method correlations (at least every 6 months)	Between all methods under same CLIA certificate (§493.1281)	Same as for CLIA	Comparison across all test sites and CLIA certificates in entire organization	Same as for CLIA

[a] All moderate-complexity requirements also apply to high-complexity test methods, but have additional requirements for personnel and method validation.

Almost immediately after publication, the EQC concept became controversial.[15] As a result, CMS currently is "rethinking EQC."[16] For now, this leaves POCT sites with three alternatives: (1) analyzing two external quality control levels per day, (2) implementing EQC after on-site evaluation, or (3) following each manufacturer's EQC approach.[17] For the future, current expectations are that CMS will modify the requirements to incorporate key concepts from CLSI guidelines currently under development to encourage test sites to develop their own quality control plan based on patient safety and risk management.[18]

Verification of performance specifications (Clinical Laboratory Improvement Amendments of 1988 sections [2003 Federal Register] §493.1253(b)) Method verification means collecting, on site, baseline data and performance data before implementing the method for routine use. The characteristics evaluated include accuracy, precision, reportable range, and reference intervals. Sites may use the manufacturer's reference ranges as long as the director determines that these are suitable for the POCT site's clientele. Verification of performance specifications is a "one-time" requirement; records must be kept for the "life" of the method plus 2 years.

Proficiency testing (Clinical Laboratory Improvement Amendments of 1988 sections [2003 Federal Register] §§493.801–865) Under CLIA, proficiency testing plays a key role in assessing test performance. Successful participation in proficiency testing is a requirement for maintaining CLIA certification for selected analytes. All sites must be enrolled in a CMS-approved proficiency testing program for those analytes identified by the CLIA regulations for which they are testing.[19] CLIA requirements identify the minimum acceptable performance criteria for successfully passing proficiency testing for each analyte in the three yearly events and mandates that proficiency testing samples be treated, as much as possible, like patient specimens. Noncompliance with proficiency testing sample handling has become a major focus for CLIA inspections. Testing sites failing the same analyte in two of three consecutive proficiency testing events can be subject to sanctions ranging from being required to submit a plan of correction to mandatory suspension of testing for the failed analyte. When POCT sites are under the central laboratory's CLIA certificate, the central laboratory participates in a CMS-approved proficiency-testing program for all regulated analytes tested. The POCT site interfaces with the proficiency testing process through method comparison data, which are collected at least semiannually as part of the quality assessment processes. If the POCT site holds its own CLIA certificate, the POCT site must participate in a CMS-approved proficiency-testing program for all regulated analytes being tested. When a proficiency-testing program is not available for an analyte, then data collected from a twice-a-year accuracy assessment (§493.1236(c)) (see below) must be collected and made available to the inspector.

Quality systems for point-of-care testing (Clinical Laboratory Improvement Amendments of 1988 subpart K [2003 Federal Register], §§493.1200–1299) Subpart K, "Quality Systems for Nonwaived Testing," a new 2003 requirement, focuses on the path of workflow for specimen analyses. It specifies the appropriate policies and procedures that must be in place to assure quality throughout the preanalytical, analytical, and postanalytical phases of the testing process. The preanalytical requirements address issues beginning with the test request and continuing through sample collection, handling, and processing. The CMS is concerned that sample integrity and positive patient identification are maintained throughout the testing process. The analytical requirements that need to be addressed include all aspects of the testing process associated with the analysis. These include the procedure manual; test system equipment, instruments, reagents, materials, and supplies; verification of performance specifications before routine implementation; maintenance and function checks; calibration and calibration verification; and quality-control procedures. Postanalytical requirements include the protocols that need to be in place to ensure accurate, reliable, and timely reporting of patient data along with the needed interpretive information on the test report.

The requirements for each of the three phases of testing emphasize quality assessment (assurance) and continuous quality improvement. The beginning of CLIA's subpart K, section §493.1200(a), states: "...establish and maintain written policies and procedures that implement and monitor a quality system for all phases of the total testing process [ie, preanalytic, analytical, and postanalytic] as well as general laboratory systems." Section §493.1200(b) goes on to state: "... quality systems must include an assessment component that ensures continuous improvement of the laboratory's [point of care] performance and services through ongoing monitoring that identifies, evaluates and resolves problems." The importance of establishing and following written polices and procedures, taking corrective actions, and making appropriate changes to prevent problems from recurring is not a new concept. With the 2003 revisions to CLIA, the emphasis of CMS has shifted even more to quality and patient safety in every step of testing.

Clearly CMS requires that testing sites continually monitor, evaluate, and improve their processes and procedures, which suggests that there are several quality requirements particularly important to a POCT site. Test results for the same analyte measured by different methodologies or instruments within the same institution and under the same certificate must be compared with each other at least twice each year (§493.1281). One effective means of accomplishing this is periodically to split specimens run at the POCT site with those at the central laboratory. The comparative results must be systematically documented and reviewed. Generally, the central laboratory is responsible for specifying the type of specimen to be used (whole blood, plasma, or quality-control material), the frequency and number of comparisons, and the criteria used for evaluating the comparison data. At least every 6 months, POCT sites must validate the accuracy of every method. This can be accomplished by proficiency testing, by analyzing samples with known concentrations, or by splitting samples with a test site known to generate quality results (ie, central or reference laboratory). Personnel competency assessment requires testing personnel to have documented training before conducting testing; furthermore, their competency must be assessed twice the first year and at least once a year thereafter for every test performed. Obviously, a POCT site, with careful planning, can use the same data for multiple purposes.

Inspection (Clinical Laboratory Improvement Amendments of 1988 sections [2003 Federal Register] §493.1773) CLIA inspects POCT sites performing moderate-complexity testing every 2 years for compliance to the regulations. Typically, inspectors are "state" employees functioning locally on CMS's behalf. A fee is assessed for this process and the inspections are unannounced.

Voluntary accreditation by professional organizations with "CMS-deemed status" (Clinical Laboratory Improvement Amendments of 1988 sections [2003 Federal Register] §493.551)
CMS allows test sites to meet all applicable CLIA requirements through accreditation by a CMS-deemed (approved), nonprofit accreditation program whose requirements are "deemed" to be equal to or more stringent than those specified in CLIA. Testing sites may choose to be accredited by a deemed organization. In 2008, approximately

207,000 testing sites received CLIA certificates; 8% of these are accredited and inspected by one of the professional accreditation organizations. CMS has the right to reinspect up to 5% of accredited testing sites.

JOINT COMMISSION

The Joint Commission (formerly known as the Joint Commission on Accreditation of Healthcare Organizations) is a voluntary organization that accredits more than 80% of United States hospitals. POCT sites in these organizations must at a minimum adhere to standards identified in the *Comprehensive Accreditation Manual for Laboratory and Point-of-Care Testing*, which is updated yearly.[4] Those standards focus on quality improvement and promotion of quality outcomes. Inspection for compliance is conducted every 2 years by inspectors hired and trained by the Joint Commission. However, the Joint Commission also accepts Cola and LAP-CAP inspections, but will reinspect test sites performing only waived testing as part of the entire organization's 3-year reaccreditation.

The Joint Commission recognizes the CLIA test complexity categories including waived test methods. The POCT sites performing waived testing and seeking Joint Commission accreditation are inspected every 2 years using the five waived testing requirements shown in **Table 3**. Each has associated "elements of performance" designed to assure safe and high-quality test results. The Joint Commission requirements for moderate-complexity testing methods generally parallel those of the CLIA and are summarized in **Table 2**.

THE LABORATORY ACCREDITATION PROGRAM OF THE COLLEGE OF AMERICAN PATHOLOGISTS

The LAP-CAP enumerates its requirements in a series of checklists.[5] All POCT sites must follow applicable standards in the Laboratory General Checklist and the Point-of-Care Testing Checklist. These are updated every 1 to 2 years and are available on the CAP Web site. Proficiency testing has long been an important component of the LAP-CAP inspection philosophy. Accredited sites must participate in proficiency testing (when available) through CAP surveys or other CAP-approved proficiency testing surveys for each analyte tested, including those tested by waived methods. The LAP-CAP emphasizes an overall total quality management approach and continuous quality improvement for the entire POCT process, including management of preanalytical, analytical, and postanalytical errors. Inspections, conducted by a trained team of "peer" laboratory professionals, are intended to be educational. Until recently, all sites were required to adhere to the same quality-testing requirements regardless of test complexity. This is no longer the case. LAP-CAP has specific requirements for waived (**Table 4**) and moderate-complexity testing (see **Table 2**).

COLA REQUIREMENTS

Cola initially focused on testing in physician office laboratories.[6] Currently it accredits many other types of test sites in a variety of clinical settings. Cola's philosophy is based on education and problem solving. Inspectors usually are medical technologists/clinical laboratory scientists who are prepared to assist test sites in meeting the regulations and generating quality test results. To prepare for the accreditation process, Cola provides sites with an initial self-inspection checklist. Inspectors use the same checklist during the on-site inspection. The requirements for both waived and moderate-complexity testing closely follow CLIA regulations. Like CMS, Cola

Table 3
Joint Commission waived testing quality requirements (2009)

Waived Testing Standard	Testing Requirement
.01.01.01	Policies and procedures for waived tests are established, current, approved, and readily available
.02.01.01	The director named on the CLIA certificate identifies the staff responsible for performing and supervising waived testing; these individuals may be employees of the organization, contracted staff, or employees of a contracted service; responsible staff may be identified within job descriptions or by listing job titles or individual names
.03.01.01	Staff and licensed independent practitioners performing waived tests are competent
.04.01.01	The [organization] performs quality control checks for waived testing on each procedure
.05.01.01	The [organization] maintains records for waived testing

Data from Laboratory accreditation standards. Joint Commission. Oakbrook Terrace (IL). Available at:http://www.jointcommission.org. Accessed December 11, 2008.

does not inspect sites performing only waived testing; requirements for moderately complex methods are summarized in **Table 2**.

POINT-OF-CARE TESTING COORDINATION

POCT is focused on providing rapid test results to improve patient outcomes. In a total quality managed environment, justification for implementing POCT should be based on objective assessments of need and analytical capabilities. Once in place, ongoing oversight is essential to ensure quality. For multiple testing sites, organizations commonly rely on a coordinator, a quality-team or -committee approach appropriate for the situation, or both.[20,21] Even standalone and limited-menu POCT programs benefit from coordination.

INDEPENDENT POINT-OF-CARE TRAINING SITES

Independent POCT sites, including those in physician office laboratories, must have their own CLIA certificate and a designated director. In addition to complying with the

Table 4
Laboratory Accreditation Program–College of American Pathologists point-of-care waived testing quality-control requirements (2007)

Waived Testing Quality-Control Requirement	Testing Requirement
POC. 07,037	Are control results documented for quantitative and qualitative tests, as applicable?
POC. 07,124	Is there evidence of corrective action when control results exceed defined tolerance limits?
POC. 07,211	Are the results of controls verified for acceptability before reporting results?

Data from Laboratory accreditation program. College of American Pathologists (CAP). Available at: http://www.cap.org/apps/cap.portal?_nfpb=true&_pagelable=accreditation. Accessed December 11, 2008.

appropriate waived and/or moderate-complexity regulations, the director under the rubric of "good laboratory practices" must consider the entire scope of operations. In the process of "directing" a POCT site, he or she must, for example, take into account the needs of clinicians using the test results; set quality standards; develop policies and procedures encompassing preanalytical, analytical, and postanalytical variables; review performance data (ie, quality control and, if appropriate, proficiency testing); and guarantee adequate staff training and competency assessment. Perhaps the most overlooked aspect of POCT is ensuring that the test results are communicated to care givers and entered into the patient's record. Typically, these wide-ranging requirements are addressed through some form of regular, director-staff interaction. A documented, 30-minute monthly staff review may be adequate.

POINT-OF-CARE TESTING SITES WITHIN HOSPITALS

Within an organization, POCT sites often are widely distributed and appear to be independent of each other and of the central laboratory. Coordination is needed to meet the requirements for a seamless, uniform testing operation across the entire organization because test results from different sites may be used to treat the same patient. Simply put, whether the organization's POCT sites have independent CLIA certificates or perform testing under the central laboratory's certificate, the quality of all test results must be independent of test site, methodology, and personnel. Oversight of POCT often falls to a designated POCT coordinator or a committee comprised of representatives from administration, the central laboratory, nursing service, clinicians, information technology, and other departments, such as pharmacy and billing. While the primary goal of coordination is to ensure that patients' needs are met, the responsibilities may include the selection of new test devices and the approval of analytes to the test menu. The CMS and the deemed-accrediting organizations recognize the importance of POCT site coordination.

REFERENCES

1. Public Law 100–578, Section 353 Public Health Service Act (42 U.S.C. 263a) October 31, 1988.
2. US Centers for Medicare & Medicaid Services (CMS). Medicare, Medicaid, and CLIA Programs: laboratory requirements relating to quality systems and certain personnel qualifications. Final rule. Current CLIA Regulations (including all changes through 01/24/2003) Available at: http://wwwn.cdc.gov/clia/regs/toc.aspx. Accessed December 11, 2008. Fed Regist 2003;16:3640–714.
3. CMS state operations manual appendix C, regulations and interpretive guidelines for laboratories and laboratory services. Available at: http://www.cms.hhs.gov/CLIA/03_Interpretive_Guidelines_for_Laboratories.aspTopOfPage. Accessed December 11, 2008.
4. Laboratory accreditation standards. Joint Commission. Oakbrook Terrace (IL). Available at: http://www.jointcommission.org. Accessed December 11, 2008.
5. Laboratory accreditation program. College of American Pathologists (CAP). Available at: http://www.cap.org/apps/cap.portal?_nfpb=true&_pageLabel=accreditation. Accessed December 11, 2008.
6. Accreditation manual. COLA. Columbia (MD). Available at: http://cola.org/. Accessed December 11, 2008.
7. CLIA certificates. Available at: http://www.cms.hhs.gov/clia/downloads/types_of_clia_certificates.pdf. Accessed December 11, 2008.

8. CLIA certificate fee schedule. Available at: http://www.cms.hhs.gov/CLIA/downloads/CLIA_certificate_fee_schedule.pdf. Accessed December 11, 2008.

9. Provider-performed microscopy procedures. Available at: http://wwwn.cdc.gov/clia/ppm.aspx. Accessed December 11, 2008.

10. CMS 116 form. Available at: http://www.cms.hhs.gov/CLIA/06_How_to_Apply_for_a_CLIA_Certificate_International_Laboratories.asp#TopOfPage. Accessed December 11, 2008.

11. Number of CLIA certificates. Available at: http://www.cms.hhs.gov/CLIA/downloads/statupda.pdf. Accessed December 11, 2008.

12. Recommendations for Clinical Laboratory Improvement Amendments of 1988 (CLIA) waiver applications for manufacturers of in vitro diagnostic devices. Available at: http://www.fda.gov/cdrh/oivd/guidance/1171.pdf. Accessed December 11, 2008.

13. CLIA test method complexity classifications. Available at: http://www.cms.hhs.gov/CLIA/10_Categorization_of_Tests.asp#TopOfPage. Accessed December 11, 2008.

14. Clinical and Laboratory Standards Institute 2008. Available at: http://www.clsi.org/. Accessed December 11, 2008.

15. Ehrmeyer SS, Laessig RH. Centers for Medicare and Medicaid Services' equivalent quality control and manufacturers' internal quality control systems: still confused after all these years? Point of Care 2008;7(2):76–8.

16. McDowell J. Revisiting equivalent quality control. Clin Lab News 2005;31(6):1,3,6.

17. Continuation and revision of the components of the Clinical Laboratory Improvement Amendments (CLIA) educational period regarding certain quality control (QC) requirements. Available at: http://www.cms.hhs.gov/SurveyCertificationGenInfo/downloads/SCLetter07-33.pdf. Accessed December 11, 2008.

18. Malone B. Risk management for clinical labs. Clin Lab News November 2008. Available at: http://www.aacc.org/publications/cln/2008/november/Pages/CovStory1Nov08.aspx. Accessed December 11, 2008.

19. CLIA proficiency testing programs. Available at: http://www.cms.hhs.gov/CLIA/downloads/ptlist.pdf. Accessed December 11, 2008.

20. Goldsmith B, Porter E. Ensuring quality in a multihospital POC program: one system's approach. Point of Care 2005;4(4):167–73.

21. Laessig RH, Ehrmeyer SS. Quality management and administration. In: Kost GJ, editor. Point-of-care testing: principles, management, and clinical practice. Philadelphia: Lippincott Williams & Wilkins; 2002. p. 422–3.

Perspectives on Cost and Outcomes for Point-of-Care Testing

Elizabeth Lee-Lewandrowski, PhD, MPH[a,b], Kent Lewandrowski, MD[b,*]

KEYWORDS
• Point-of-care testing • Cost • Outcomes

PERSPECTIVES ON COST

It is generally perceived that point-of-care testing (POCT) is more expensive on a unit-cost basis than testing performed in a centralized laboratory.[1–7] This concept reflects the fact that the cost of consumables for POCT is typically greater than it is for tests performed using automated laboratory instruments and the fact that point-of-care tests are performed one at a time and, therefore, cannot achieve the economy of scale afforded by high-volume automated testing. Various studies have compared the cost of POCT to that of central laboratory tests, as summarized by Foster and colleagues (**Table 1**).[2] Although most studies indicate that POCT is more expensive than central laboratory testing, that is not always the case. Some studies have shown that POCT is not invariably more expensive, depending on the test volume, testing technology, program management, and other factors.[3] In one study, Bailey and colleagues[8] reported an institutional savings of $392,336, with a reduction in unit cost from $15.33 per panel to $8.03, following institution-wide implementation of POCT for blood gases and electrolytes.

Despite a significant volume of literature on this subject, calculating the actual cost of POCT compared with that of the central laboratory remains an enigma. Unit cost reflects only one part of the overall equation. Other factors must also be considered, as summarized in article by Lewandrowski.[9] These include the impact of reduced turnaround time on the time to diagnosis and treatment, impact of testing on the overall cost of care, issues of workflow on clinical units, impact on test use, length of patient stay, and potential improvements to clinical outcomes. Lacking a clear consensus in the literature, the decision of whether to implement POCT or use a central laboratory

[a] Research Core Laboratory, Massachusetts General Hospital, 55 Fruit Street, Gray 5 Chemistry, Boston, MA 02114, USA
[b] Department of Pathology, Massachusetts General Hospital, Harvard Medical School, 55 Fruit Street, Gray 5 Chemistry, Boston, MA 02114, USA
* Corresponding author.
E-mail address: klewandrowski@partners.org (K. Lewandrowski).

Clin Lab Med 29 (2009) 479–489
doi:10.1016/j.cll.2009.07.001
0272-2712/09/$ – see front matter © 2009 Published by Elsevier Inc.

labmed.theclinics.com

Table 1
Selected cost comparisons between POCT and central laboratory testing (in US dollars)

Tests	POCT Cost	Central Laboratory Testing Cost	Reference
Glucose	$11.50	$3.19	3
	$6.62	$3.30	4
	$7.12	$6.85	5
Blood gases/electrolyes	$45.00	$9.50	5
Chemistry and hematocrit	$14.37–16.67	$20.62	6
Mixed emergency department menu	$19.20	$2.94	7

Data from Foster K, Despotis G, Scott M. Point-of-care testing. Cost issues and impact on hospital operations. In: Lewandrowski K, guest editor. Point of care testing. Clinics in Laboratory Medicine, vol. 21, no. 2. Clin Lad Med 2001;21:269–84.

will depend on a number of factors beyond unit cost. Many of these factors are unique to the individual hospital or care unit.

One of the issues related to unit-cost analysis for POCT concerns the conceptual model for determining labor costs. In contrast, the cost of consumables is usually straightforward. In calculating labor costs for central laboratory testing, one must include in-laboratory labor costs and preanalytic labor costs for services such as phlebotomy and nursing (**Table 2**). To obtain a central laboratory test, phlebotomy supplies must first be gathered, a requisition (or order entry) test request must be completed, tubes must be labeled, and the sample specimen must be collected. The specimen must then be packaged and sent to the laboratory, either by pneumatic tube or by human courier. After the sample is in the laboratory, the test request must be accessioned (or, in the case of order entry, receipt acknowledged), the specimen must then be processed, and the testing performed. In contrast, using POCT, supplies must be gathered, the specimen collected, and the test performed. In this model, POCT eliminates many of the preanalytic steps, all of which involve labor cost. Calculating the actual labor cost requires a detailed time-and-motion study and must take

Table 2
Hypothetical labor steps involved in central laboratory testing versus POCT

Steps	Central Laboratory Testing	POCT
Order test	X	X
Acknowledge order	X	X
Label tubes or other consumables	X	X
Collect specimen	X	X
Package specimen	X	—
Transport specimen	X	—
Receive and acknowledge receipt (or accession)	X	—
Process specimen	X	—
Perform test	X	X
Release result	X	—
Receive result	X	X

into consideration differential hourly rates for phlebotomists, nurses, and medical technologists. Conceptually, the POCT labor model can be significantly less expensive than the cost for all of the labor-consuming steps that are involved in the central laboratory model. However, each test is different and each clinical situation unique. It is therefore not possible to make generalizations about the labor-cost model for POCT compared with the central laboratory model.

The central concept underlying the justification for POCT is turnaround time. The presumption is that faster turnaround time is necessarily better for patient care and for hospital operations. However, in many situations this is not the case. More to the point, test results must be made available in a clinically relevant time frame. For example, the use of whole-blood cardiac-marker POCT testing in the emergency department permits physicians to make rapid decisions concerning triage, diagnosis, and disposition for patients who have acute coronary syndromes. This may facilitate the making of treatment decisions and allow for efficient disposition of the patient to the appropriate hospital setting (eg, observation unit, catheterization laboratory, cardiac intensive care unit). As an alternate example, prostate-specific antigen (PSA) testing is commonly used in outpatient settings to screen for prostate cancer. Usually this test is co-ordered with other screening tests such as cholesterol and fasting plasma glucose as part of the routine health assessment. Implementing a point-of-care test for PSA in a primary care setting would be costly and would not appreciably alter clinical care or physician practice efficiency unless all of the screening tests were made available at the time of the office visit. On the other hand, implementing POCT for hemoglobin A1c in a diabetes clinic setting could potentially allow for immediate adjustments to the patient's diabetic care during the office visit, regardless of what other tests may have been ordered.

There are some tests that, regardless of cost, must be performed at the point of care. An example is the activated clotting-time test. This test (described further in the article by Van Cott in this issue) is used to monitor high-dose heparin therapy in patients who are undergoing cardiac surgery, interventional radiological procedures, extracorporeal membrane oxygenation, and other procedures. After the sample is collected, the blood immediately begins to clot. There is no time for transport to a central laboratory. Another common example is provider-performed microscopy that involves potassium hydroxide preparations in outpatient settings that are removed from a central laboratory. As one final example, rapid influenza testing can be used to identify patients who may benefit from antiviral therapy. These antibiotics must be administered very early in the course of infection to reduce the patient's symptomatic interval. Few central laboratories offer around-the-clock influenza testing. In many outpatient clinics, the time required for transport to a central laboratory is impractical to allow for timely decisions concerning antiviral therapy.

When compared with the cost of many heath care services, laboratory testing is inexpensive. It is generally recognized that laboratory testing comprises only about 4% of the average hospital budget. Yet laboratory testing directly impacts nearly two thirds of hospital activities and the cost associated with this care. Viewed in this perspective, laboratory testing should be seen as an enabling technology that can improve (or impair) the efficiency and quality of patient care. When considering whether to implement POCT, it is important to consider unit cost compared with unit value. An expensive test such as a rapid cardiac troponin test that can influence medical decision making or improve the efficiency of clinical operations may be highly cost effective.[7] Conversely, an inexpensive test for troponin that is too slow may negatively impact care and result in inefficient use of expensive hospital capacity. The rapid troponin test has a high unit value, whereas the slow but inexpensive test is essentially worthless. As one final example, POCT for creatinine is being increasingly used in radiology departments to evaluate renal function in patients before administering contrast agents for CT scans. Patients who have impaired renal function, as reflected by an abnormal estimated glomerular filtration rate, are at increased risk for contrast-induced acute kidney injury. Screening patients at the point of care permits rapid decisions to be made concerning which patients need appropriate preventive measures and promotes more efficient use of highly expensive CT scanners. If the same test were sent to the clinical laboratory, CT scans might be significantly delayed. The CT scanner would stand idle, resulting in inefficient use of expensive CT capacity.

PERSPECTIVES ON OUTCOMES

Because POCT is generally more expensive than central laboratory testing and may be difficult to manage from a regulatory perspective, it is important when considering implementation of POCT to document that some positive impact has been achieved. In other words, you need to show that the testing actually accomplishes something useful to justify the increased incremental cost. The term generally used for this is "outcomes." Outcomes may take several forms, as shown in **Table 3**. In the authors' experience, there are different types of outcomes. First, there are medical outcomes. These outcomes are reflected in data on morbidity and mortality. The patient lives longer, has fewer complications, or shows other improvements in his or her medical condition. In the authors' experience, these types of outcomes can be very difficult to document. Often, studies on medical outcomes require large numbers of patients and long follow-up. As an example of this problem, consider that with all of the research that has been performed on PSA screening and mammography, there is, as yet, only inconclusive evidence that the screenings actually improve long-term survival. In some cases, performing controlled outcomes studies would be ethically questionable because patients could be denied laboratory testing that is part of the established standard of care.

Then there are financial outcomes. In theory, these should be easy to document if one applies a robust cost accounting system. In practice, however, the task is not so easy. Medical care involves a complex interaction of a large number of variables, each of which influence the others in sometimes poorly understood ways. In isolation, one can add up the cost of testing reagents and labor and assign a value for overhead to determine which test, point-of-care or central laboratory, is more expensive. However, such analysis does not take into consideration the possible impact of

Table 3
Classification of clinical outcomes

Types of Outcome	Examples/Comments
Medical outcomes	Decreased morbidity or mortality, improved functional status. May be difficult to document. May require long-term follow-up of large numbers of patients.
Financial outcomes	Decreased cost or cost avoidance. May appear to be straightforward to document, but in practice most financial outcomes rely on highly artificial cost accounting models.
Operational outcomes	Decreased hospital length of stay, improved capacity use. Usually not difficult to document. Many operational parameters are already routinely monitored by hospitals.

a more rapid test result on medical decisions, patient outcomes, hospital operations, differential reimbursement rates, and other factors. As a consequence, most cost analyses that the authors have observed concerning laboratory testing, including those that they have published, are highly artificial and are, for practical purposes, essentially worthless.

Finally there are operational outcomes. These include metrics such as length of stay, throughput, and other measures of efficiency. These are usually not too difficult to measure, and in fact, most hospitals perform these measurements routinely as part of clinical operations dashboards. In the case of POCT, it is not difficult to measure, for example, emergency department length of stay before and after implementation of a new test.[1,7,10] Indeed, there is only modest and selective evidence in the literature that POCT as opposed to central laboratory testing improves clinical outcomes. However, there is abundant evidence that POCT can improve efficiency and hospital operations.

An important consideration when evaluating the impact of POCT on outcomes is to evaluate whether the outcome simply resulted from the availability of a new test or whether it resulted specifically from implementation of POCT. For example, Mueller and colleagues[11] reported on a prospective, randomized, controlled study of 452 patients who presented to the emergency department with dyspnea. Patients were assigned to a diagnostic strategy using a point-of-care B-type natriuretic peptide assay or to standard care without natriuretic peptide testing. The time to discharge and the total cost of treatment were evaluated. The study demonstrated that the patients who received POCT natriuretic peptide testing had a decreased hospital length of stay (8 days versus 11 days) and a decreased total cost of care ($5,410 versus $7,264). Presumably, these outcomes resulted from the ability of the POCT test to provide a rapid diagnosis and allow for earlier commencement of appropriate treatment for patients in that group compared with the patients that did not receive natriuretic peptide testing. In a separate study, Green and colleagues[12] evaluated hospital length of stay, postdischarge mortality, and rates of rehospitalization following implementation of N-terminal prohormone brain nutriuretic peptide (NT-proBNP) testing in the central laboratory. They documented a decrease in hospital length of stay of 1.86 days, a decrease in postdischarge 60-day mortality, and a decrease in the rate of rehospitalization. The question then remains, were the outcomes the result of POCT or were the outcomes the result of making natriuretic testing available, either in the central laboratory or at the point of care. Another example of this dilemma concerns the use of fecal occult blood testing (FOBT) to screen for colorectal carcinoma. There is clear evidence that the appropriate use of FOBT can reduce mortality from colorectal cancer (see the article on FOBT by Sanford & McPherson in this issue). FOBT can be performed in the home, the physician's office, or a central laboratory. There is no clinical or operational need for rapid testing. Rather, it is important that the test is performed, that the results are followed up, and that the test be done properly according to established guidelines. Although FOBT is often considered a point-of-care test, the performance of this test at the point of care offers no real advantage.

Given the previous discussion and the nuances described when evaluating outcomes, it is useful to consider cases in which there is good evidence to indicate that improved outcomes resulted from the implementation of POCT (**Table 4**). Selected examples are described in this article, and some of them are discussed further in other articles by Sanford & McPherson, Lewandrowski, Alter & Deines and Campbell in this issue. Previous publications regarding POCT and outcomes provide augmentation of this discussion.[13–15] Of particular note, the reader is referred to article

Table 4
Selected examples of improved outcomes resulting from POCT

Tests	Outcomes/Comments
1. Patient home capillary-glucose monitoring test	Permits tight glycemic control with associated improved outcomes.
2. Tight glycemic control in intensive care settings	Improved outcomes in intensive care settings (see article in this issue by [first author's name] on tight glycemic control).
3. Patient home self-monitoring of anticoagulation	Documented improvements to maintaining appropriate level of long-term anticoagulation.
4. POCT cardiac markers in the emergency department	Multiple studies show reduced emergency department length of stay.
5. POCT D-dimer test in the emergency department	Decreased emergency department length of stay and increased rate of discharges to home.
6. POCT rapid urine drugs-of-abuse test	Decreased emergency department length of stay.
7. Rapid influenza test	Facilitates early antiviral therapy.
8. Rapid HIV test in emergency departments and outpatient clinics	Facilitates identification of HIV infection and improves rate of appropriate follow-up.
9. Intraoperative parathyroid hormone test	Improved success of parathyroid surgery.

by Nichols and colleagues.[13] which includes a comprehensive evidence-based discussion of a number of point-of-care technologies.

Home Self-Testing of Capillary Glucose in Patients who have Diabetes Mellitus

Capillary blood glucose tests originally gained popularity as a means for patients who have diabetes to self-monitor their own glucose levels. These technologies revolutionized diabetes care, permitting patients to maintain tight glycemic control. They have been clearly linked to improved outcomes in terms of retinopathy, nephropathy, and certain vascular complications.

Tight Glycemic Control in Intensive Care Settings

This topic is covered in detail in the article by Alter & Deines in this issue.

Patient Home Self-Monitoring of Anticoagulation

Patient self-testing to monitor Coumadin therapy was, for a number of years, highly controversial. Laboratory professionals were concerned that self-testing for prothrombin time was potentially dangerous and that the devices were unreliable compared with tests performed in the central laboratory. Subsequent studies have shown that with proper training and more reliable devices, patients can achieve better anticoagulation management using self-testing as opposed to being monitored exclusively in the physician's office. This topic is discussed further in the article Van Cott in this issue.

POCT for Cardiac Markers in the Emergency Department

Several studies have documented that the performance of rapid, whole-blood, cardiac-marker testing (eg, for troponin, creatine kinase-MB, myoglobin) may result in a decrease in either emergency department or hospital length of stay (**Table 5**).[16–18] This topic was recently reviewed by Storrow.[18] Virtually all studies have shown significant reductions in test turnaround time, which is, itself, an outcome. However, reduced turnaround time is only helpful if it is associated with improved patient care, financial improvements, or improved efficiency of clinical operations (such as decreased emergency department length of stay). One result of these studies is that an increasing number of hospitals are implementing rapid, whole-blood, cardiac-marker testing in the emergency department. However, it is noteworthy that no published studies to date have documented cases of patients who had acute coronary syndromes for whom improved clinical outcomes resulted from the implementation of rapid cardiac marker testing at the point of care. The clinical justification for rapid cardiac-marker testing is discussed further in the article on cardiac markers by Lewandrowski in this issue.

POCT for B-type natriuretic peptides has also been shown to reduce hospital length of stay, but as with a previous discussion in this article, it is not clear that this outcome resulted from simply making the new test available, regardless of whether it was performed in a central laboratory or at the point of care.

POCT for D-Dimer to rule out Deep-Venous Thrombosis and Pulmonary Embolism

D-dimer is a protein product of fibrinolysis that can be measured in the blood. When a blood clot forms, the fibrinolysis system is activated to begin removal of the clot. One component of this system is the enzyme plasmin, which digests fibrin in the clot, producing fibrin fragments in the blood. One of these fragments is D-dimer. An elevated level of D-dimer indicates that fibrinolysis is occurring and, by inference, that a clot is present. In patients who have deep-venous thrombosis (DVT) or pulmonary embolism (PE), the D-dimer level is typically elevated. The D-dimer test is not specific for DVT or PE, however, because there are other causes for an elevated D-dimer level such as disseminated intravascular coagulation and liver disease. One of the cornerstones in the approach to a patient who has a possible DVT is the concept of risk stratification to determine the pretest probability of a DVT (see **Fig. 1**). The most commonly used system is the Well's Score. This system assigns points for various risk factors for DVT, such as cancer, immobilization, and edema of a single leg. The points are added to assign the patient into a low-, moderate-, or high-risk category. In low-risk patients, the appropriate first step is to test for the presence of D-dimer. If

---

Table 5
Studies documenting improved outcomes resulting from POCT for cardiac markers in the emergency department

Studies (Year)	Outcomes
Apple (2006)[16]	Decreased hospital length of stay of 4 hours
Lee-Lewandrowski (2001)[7]	Decreased emergency department length of stay of 47 minutes. Increased rate of discharge of patients who had chest pain.
Singer (2005)[17]	Decreased emergency department length of stay of 1.9 hours.

Data from Storrow A. A systematic review of emergency department point-of-care cardiac markers and ED efficiency measures. Point of Care, in press.

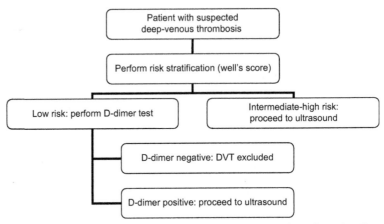

Fig. 1. Approach to the patient who has suspected deep-venous thrombosis (DVT).

the D-dimer test is negative, that finding will essentially exclude the diagnosis of DVT. If the test is positive, then an ultrasound is required to confirm the diagnosis. Moderate- and high-risk patients require an ultrasound regardless of the D-dimer value. For these patients, D-dimer testing is unnecessary before ultrasound procedures are performed. The approach for the patient who has a suspected PE is very similar. The first step is to perform a risk stratification to determine the pretest probability of a PE. Patients are divided in low-, moderate- and high-risk categories. Low-risk patients should be tested for the presence of D-dimer. If the D-dimer test is negative, then the diagnosis of PE can be essentially excluded. If the test is positive, then a CT scan or other study should be performed to confirm the diagnosis. Moderate- to high-risk patients should receive a CT scan regardless of the D-dimer value. Therefore, in the evaluation of possible DVT or PE, D-dimer testing is primarily useful for the exclusion of a diagnosis of DVT or PE in low-risk patients. Positive results must be confirmed using the appropriate radiologic study. The D-dimer test is of little value in moderate- to high-risk patients, who always require radiologic scans. Conceptually, the D-dimer test should help to reduce the use of unnecessary and expensive ultrasound and CT scans. Used appropriately, the test is highly cost effective.

One recent study reported on the implementation of a rapid, whole-blood, D-dimer test in the emergency department.[1] After implementation, the mean and median length of stay in the emergency department was significantly reduced for patients who received the rapid, D-dimer, point-of-care test. Another outcome that was demonstrated was a change in patient disposition. With the rapid test, fewer patients were admitted and a higher percentage was discharged home from the emergency department. There was also an increase in patients who were admitted to a short-stay observation unit, presumably at the expense of regular hospital admissions. Interestingly, there was no significant change in the use of radiologic testing after implementation of the test.

The experience with rapid POCT for cardiac markers and D-dimer illustrates an important concept concerning outcomes and POCT. Not all forms of POCT in the emergency department have been shown to improve patient care or emergency department operations. For example, two studies evaluated POCT for common, routine analytes (eg, electrolytes, blood gases, hematocrit) in the emergency department.[19,20] In both studies, laboratory test turnaround time was significantly reduced, but there was no demonstrable impact on emergency department length of stay. The important difference between the menu of tests used in those studies as opposed to tests for cardiac markers and D-dimer is that the latter two tests directly impact a key point in decision making concerning triage, diagnosis, or disposition, as shown in **Fig. 1**. In contrast, performing a small number of routine chemistry tests is ineffective because those tests do not directly affect key decision steps in the evaluation of emergency room patients. Furthermore, in regard to tests of blood gases and electrolytes, in most cases, other routine tests such as a complete blood count or liver function are co-ordered with those tests. Accomplishing a rapid turnaround time for some, but not all, of those tests would usually have minimal impact on emergency department length of stay.

POCT for Urine Drugs of Abuse in the Emergency Department

A recent study evaluated the impact of implementation of rapid urine drugs-of-abuse testing in the emergency department.[10] In that study, a decrease in the mean and median length of stay in the emergency department was documented. One unique feature of the study site was that the emergency department included a large acute psychiatric service. Drugs-of-abuse testing was performed as one component of the protocol to medically clear patients before admission or discharge to an outpatient care setting.

POCT for Influenza A and B

This topic was discussed previously in this article and is discussed in the article by Lewandrowski in this issue.

Rapid POCT for HIV Infection

Several manufacturers have marketed rapid point-of-care HIV tests that use either blood or salivary samples. This topic is discussed in more detail in the article by Campbell in this issue. There are three settings in which these tests have been employed:

A. Employee needle-stick (sharp) injuries: Hospital employees may be put at risk for occupational HIV infection resulting from needle-stick injuries from infected patients. A key component of managing these cases is to decide whether to administer prophylactic antiretroviral drug therapy to the employee. This decision may be guided by testing the patient for HIV antibodies. Most hospital laboratories are not equipped to offer timely HIV testing on a 24-hour basis. In such a situation, rapid HIV tests may be employed.

B. Rapid point-of-care HIV testing in outpatient clinics and emergency departments: A significant number of patients who are infected with HIV are unaware of their infection. Some of these patients lack heath insurance, are indigent, or are otherwise at risk for being lost to medical follow-up after HIV testing. When testing is performed in a central clinical laboratory, the test results typically are not available until after the patient has left the clinic or emergency department. Implementation of POCT for HIV permits results to be made available before the patient has left the clinical facility. Presumably this allows patients to be set up with outpatient HIV treatment resources before they are lost to follow-up.

C. Rapid HIV testing in pregnant patients presenting in labor but without prenatal care: In patients presenting in labor who have had no prenatal care, there is potential risk for maternal–fetal HIV transmission during delivery. In an HIV-infected mother, the risk for transmission can be significantly reduced by administration of antiretroviral prophylaxis. The decision to administer these drugs can be guided by using rapid HIV testing.

POCT to Monitor Hemostasis in Surgical Patients

The potential utility of POCT for intraoperative hemostasis monitoring of patients during cardiopulmonary bypass was reviewed by Despotis and colleagues.[21] Such patients are at increased risk for excessive perioperative blood loss that may necessitate the transfusion of blood products. POCT can facilitate patient-specific adjustment of heparin and protamine dosing, resulting in reduced blood loss and need for transfusions.

SUMMARY

POCT is usually more expensive on a unit-cost basis than testing performed in a central laboratory. POCT is also notoriously difficult to manage, and it is challenging to maintain regulatory compliance for POCT, especially in large institutions. For these reasons, it is important to demonstrate that POCT can improve patient outcomes or clinical operational efficiency before testing is implemented. Although the literature on POCT and its relationship to improved outcomes is not extensive, some POCT technologies have been shown to improve patient outcomes (eg, patient self-glucose monitoring in the home, tight glycemic control in intensive care settings) or to improve hospital or emergency department operations (eg, whole-blood cardiac-marker testing and D-dimer testing in the emergency department). In some cases, these outcomes result simply by making a new test available rather than by being a direct consequence of performing testing at the point of care. However, in most cases, the rapid turnaround time provided by POCT is the main factor that is ultimately responsible for the improvement in outcomes.

REFERENCES

1. Lewandrowski E, Nichols J, Van Cott E, et al. Implementation of a rapid whole blood D-dimer test in the emergency department of an urban academic medical center: impact on ED length of stay and ancillary test utilization. Am J Clin Pathol, in press.
2. Foster K, Despotis G, Scott M. Point-of-care testing. Cost issues and impact on hospital operations. In: Lewandrowski K, guest editor. Point of care testing. Clinics in laboratory medicine, Vol. 21, no. 2. St. Louis (MO): Elsevier Saunders; 2001. p. 269–84.
3. Lewandrowski E, Laposata M, Eschenbach K, et al. Utilization and cost analysis of bedside capillary glucose testing in a large teaching hospital: implications for the management of point of care testing. Am J Med 1994;97:222–30.
4. Winkelman J, Wybenga D, Tanasijevic M. The fiscal consequences of central vs. distributed testing of glucose. Clin Chem 1994;40:1628–30.
5. Nosanchuk J, Keefner R. Cost analysis of point-of-care laboratory testing in a community hospital. Am J Clin Pathol 1995;103:240–3.
6. Tsai W, Nash D, Seamonds B, et al. Point-of-care versus central laboratory testing: an ecomonic analysis in an academic medical center. Clin Ther 1995;16:898–910.
7. Lee-Lewandrowski E, Corboy D, Lewandrowski K, et al. Implementation of a point of care satellite laboratory in the emergency department of an academic medical center: impact on test turnaround time and patient length of stay. Arch Pathol Lab Med 2003;127:456–60.

8. Bailey TM, Topham TM, Wantz S, et al. Laboratory process improvement through point-of-care testing. Jt Comm J Qual Improv 1997;23(7):362–80.

9. Lewandrowski K. Point-of-care testing: an overview and look to the future. In: Lewandrowski K, guest editor. Point of care testing. Clinics in laboratory medicine, Vol. 21, no. 2. St Louis (MO): Elsevier Saunders; 2001. p. 217–39.

10. Lewandrowski K, Flood J, Finn C, et al. Implementation of point-of-care rapid urine drugs of abuse testing in the emergency department of an academic medical center: impact on test utilization and ED length of stay. Am J Clin Pathol 2008;129:796–801.

11. Mueller C, Scholer A, Laule-Lilian K, et al. Use of B-type natriuretic peptide in the evaluation and management of acute dyspnea. N Engl J Med 2004;350:647–54.

12. Green S, Redmond P, Januzzi J, et al. The impact of amino-terminal pro-brain natriuretic peptide testing on hospital length of stay and morbidity in patients with acute decompensated heart failure. Arch Pathol Lab Med 2007;131:473–6.

13. Nichols J, Christenson R, Gronowski A, et al. Executive summary. The National Academy of Clinical Biochemistry Laboratory Medicine Practice Guideline: evidence-based practice for point-of-care testing. Clin Chim Acta 2007;379: 14–28.

14. Price C, Hicks J, editors. Point of care testing. 1st edition. Washington, DC: AACC Press; 1999.

15. Lewandrowski K, guest editor. Point of care testing. Clinics in laboratory medicine, Vol. 21, no. 2. St Louis (MO): Elsevier Saunders; 2001.

16. Apple F, Chung A, Kogut M, et al. Decreased patient charges following implementation of point-of-care cardiac troponin monitoring in acute coronary syndrome patients in a community hospital cardiology unit. Clin Chim Acta 2006;370:191–5.

17. Singer A, Ardise J, Gula J, et al. Point-of-care testing reduces length of stay in emergency department chest pain patients. Ann Emerg Med 2005;45:587–91.

18. Storrow A. A systematic review of emergency department point-of-care cardiac markers and ED efficiency measures. Point of Care, in press.

19. Kendall J, Reeves B, Clancey M. Point-of-care testing: a randomized, controlled trial of clinical outcome. BMJ 1998;316:1052–7.

20. Parvin C, Lo S, Deuser S, et al. Impact of point-of-care testing on patient's length of stay in a large emergency department. Clin Chem 1996;42:711–7.

21. Despotis G, Joist J, Goodnough L. Monitoring of hemostasis in cardiac surgical patients: impact of point-of-care testing on blood loss and transfusion outcomes. Clin Chem 1997;43:1684–96.

HIV Testing Near the Patient: Changing the Face of HIV Testing

Sheldon Campbell, MD, PhD[a],*, Yuri Fedoriw, MD[b]

KEYWORDS

- Human immunodeficiency virus • Pointrop-care
- Rapid testing • Diagnostic protocol • HIV antibody tests
- HIV diagnostic algorithms

Of the approximately 1 million people infected with HIV in the United States, approximately a quarter are unaware of their serostatus;[1] worldwide, several studies in sub-Saharan Africa suggest that only about 12% of men and 10% of women know their HIV status, while in maternal health, a mere 10% of women in sub-Saharan Africa are tested for HIV.[2]

This sero-unaware population plays a major role in the incidence of new HIV cases.[3–6] Patients with limited access to health care systems and social services likely represent a significant population participating in ongoing transmission.[5] Since the early 1980s, net HIV infections and AIDS diagnoses in the developed world have decreased significantly thanks in part to risk-based screening, sensitive and specific HIV-testing methods, counseling, and the advent of highly active antiretroviral therapy (HAART). However, the rate of decline has leveled off, most likely because of the time-course of the infection and inefficiencies in the diagnosis, prevention, and treatment of new infections. Conventional testing protocols have drawbacks, one of the most important of which is the time it takes for results. That can be a matter of days or even weeks. Delay in reporting HIV test results profoundly affects the health care system, resulting in delayed and missed diagnosis and in management errors. Patients suffer anxiety and inconvenience as well.[7] Over the past decade, these concerns have fueled the development of rapid HIV tests, which are reshaping diagnostic protocols and screening recommendations.[8–11] Rapid HIV tests are being used both in the clinical laboratory and at the point of care, and may become available for home use.[12,13] As experience is gained with rapid testing, and as evolving testing recommendations are incorporated into practice, previously neglected populations can be targeted, and circumstances where immediate results will change patient

[a] Department of Laboratory Medicine, Yale University School of Medicine, New Haven, CT 06520, USA
[b] Department of Pathology and Laboratory Medicine, Division of Hematopathology, University of North Carolina, CB # 7525, School of Medicine Campus, Chapel Hill, NC 27599, USA
* Corresponding author.
E-mail address: sheldon.campbell@yale.edu (S. Campbell).

Clin Lab Med 29 (2009) 491–501
doi:10.1016/j.cll.2009.06.011
0272-2712/09/$ – see front matter. Published by Elsevier Inc.

labmed.theclinics.com

care can be addressed. This review summarizes rapid HIV tests and their use near the patient to improve access and quality of care.

PERFORMANCE OF RAPID HIV TESTS

Currently, six rapid HIV tests are approved by the US Food and Drug Administration (FDA) for clinical use (**Table 1**): OraQuick Advance (OraSure Technologies, Bethlehem, Pennsylvania), Uni-Gold Recombigen (Trinity Biotech USA, Jamestown, New York), Reveal G3 (MedMira, Inc, Halifax, Nova Scotia, Canada), Multispot (Bio-Rad Laboratories, Redmond, Washington), and two recently approved systems from Chembio, the Clearview HIV 1/2 STAT-PAK, and Clearview Complete HIV 1/2 (Chembio Diagnostic Systems, Inc, Medford, New York). Each is based on immunochemical methods in which antibody-target antigen interactions produce a colorimetric result. The Clearview assays employ identical immunochromatographic test strips and differ only in user interface. Two of the assays, Uni-Gold Recombigen and Reveal G3, are not approved for the detection of HIV-2, and Multispot stands alone among the rapid assays in its ability to not only detect, but also to differentiate HIV-1 from HIV-2 infection. In addition, the performance of a first-generation rapid HIV-1 assay, the Single Use Diagnostic System HIV-1 (Abbott Laboratories, Abbott Park, Illinois) was extensively studied before its removal from clinical use. The information gleaned from these studies and from those involving current methods describes the role of rapid HIV assays in decreasing HIV transmission and improving HIV care. As new testing protocols and strategies are being defined, other tests are being studied and will certainly be subjects of approval applications soon.[13]

The FDA data[14–18] using various seroconversion panels and known positive and negative control samples document the excellent performance characteristics of the rapid tests with sensitivity and specificity comparable to conventional enzyme immunoassays. The analogous sensitivity to conventional methods is somewhat surprising given the narrow range of antigens targeted by these assays. In fact, two of the approved assays, the Multispot and the OraQuick systems exclusively identify antibodies to HIV-1 gp41, while the remaining systems (Uni-Gold Recombigen, Reveal G3, and both Clearview systems) include only one additional antigenic target, gp120. One study addresses the limited antigenic suites demonstrating a negative OraQuick result in a series of patients treated with HAART after known HIV exposure with low viral load and decreasing gp41 antibody response.[19] This patient population would be unlikely to be followed with rapid HIV testing by current practice, and the addition of gp120 as an antigenic target may accurately identify infected patients in this setting. However, no comprehensive studies have been published that characterize the limitations of these rapid assays in relevant clinical scenarios, namely in regard to their potential use in two-stage confirmatory testing protocols.

While in most cases the rapid tests appear to have similar performance, one study found differences in sensitivity of rapid tests in early HIV infection.[20] A panel of plasma samples from recently infected individuals was tested with rapid methods, laboratory-based enzyme immunoassays, and nucleic acid amplification testing (NAAT). Of the samples, 42 were negative for HIV antibody by at least one screening test but were NAAT-positive. Fourteen of the 42 were positive with Genetic Systems HIV-1/HIV-2 PLUS O enzyme immunoassay, a third-generation test, but none of the 42 was reactive with the first-generation Vironostika HIV-1 Microelisa (bioMerieux, Inc, Durham, North Carolina). Of the four rapid tests studied, OraQuick and Clearview each detected 1 of 42 NAAT-positive samples. The Uni-Gold test, however, was positive in 11 of 42, and the Multispot was positive in 7 of 42. Of the 42 tested samples, 30 of

Table 1
FDA-approved rapid HIV tests

Test Name	Manufacturer	Specimen Type	Clinical Laboratories Improvement Amendment Category	Equipment Required	List Price	Antigens Represented
OraQuick Advance Rapid HIV-1/2 Antibody Test	OraSure Technologies, Inc	Whole blood, oral fluid, plasma	Waived; moderate complexity	Timer	$17.50	gp41
Reveal G3, Rapid HIV-1 Antibody Test	MedMira, Inc	Serum, plasma	Moderate complexity	Centrifuge, refrigerator	$14.00	gp41, gp120
Uni-Gold Recombigen HIV Test	Trinity BioTech	Whole blood, serum, plasma	Waived; moderate complexity	Timer	$15.75	gp41, gp120
Multispot HIV-1/HIV-2 RapidTest	Bio-Rad Laboratories	Serum, plasma	Moderate complexity	Centrifuge, refrigerator, laboratory equipment	$25.00	gp41
Clearview HIV 1/2 Stat Pak	Chembio Diagnostic Systems, Inc	Whole blood, serum, plasma	Waived; moderate complexity	Timer	$17.50	gp41, gp120
Clearview Complete HIV 1/2	Chembio Diagnostic Systems, Inc	Whole blood, serum, plasma	Moderate complexity	Timer	$18.50	gp41, gp120

Data from Centers for Disease Control and Prevention (http://www.cdc.gov/hiv/topics/testing/rapid/rt-purchasing.htm and http://www.cdc.gov/hiv/topics/testing/rapid/rt-comparison.htm), manufacturers' package inserts, and Food and Drug Administration.

the 42 patients had follow-up samples available. All were positive by Uni-Gold and Multispot; 26 of 30 were positive by OraQuick; and 29 of 30 were positive by the Clearview system. In discussing the findings of this study, investigators noted that the Uni-Gold uses a sandwich-capture format and may detect IgM better than other rapids. It also uses significantly more blood, which might be problematic in some settings.

USE OF RAPID TESTS FOR CONFIRMATION OR FINAL DIAGNOSIS

As for most simple immunoassays, nonspecific reactivity and other factors can generate false-positive rapid test results. For ideal application of rapid tests in outreach settings, an equally rapid confirmatory method would be ideal. A second rapid test has been used as a confirmatory method in a small number of publications with promising results.[21–23] However, no large randomized trial has examined this strategy, and it is possible that publication bias affects this literature.

In December 2007, a conference was convened to

...facilitate presentation and discussion on the performance and applications of proposed HIV test algorithms drafted by Association of Public Health Laboratories and Centers for Disease Control and Prevention (APHL/CDC) workgroups. The goal of the conference was to provide information for the development of APHL/CDC guidelines on the combinations of assays that can be used to aid in the diagnosis of HIV-1 and/or HIV-2 infection in community, clinical, and laboratory settings in the United States.

New York state and New Jersey public health testing programs reported that high percentages of clients with reactive rapid test results (25.7%[24] and 25.8%[25] respectively) failed to return for confirmatory test results. The possibility that a system of rapid tests could provide more immediate testing with greater confidence is potentially important. Several presentations at this conference addressed the use of testing algorithms designed for use at the point of care.

A study in an emergency room population[26] involved 1539 patients, 5 of whom had positive initial screening tests. Of the 5, 4 were positive with a second rapid test; all 4 were Western blot–positive, while the remaining patient was Western blot–negative.

The New Jersey Department of Public Health (NJDPH) Laboratory tested samples from 363 individuals with initially reactive rapid tests in the field.[25] The specimens were tested with additional rapid tests as well as with Western blots. Of these, 355 (97.8%) were reactive by all the other rapid tests; each of these was confirmed positive by Western. The remaining 8 (2.2%) initially positive specimens were negative by the other rapid tests and also by Western blot. Repeated testing of those 8 specimens with the initial screening test remained reactive, reinforcing the value of a second, supplementary, rapid test.

The CDC modeled the performance of various point-of-care algorithms using data from a prospective evaluation of FDA-approved rapid tests.[27] A two-test algorithm was almost always able to distinguish true-positive from false-positive screening tests. Modeling suggested that adding a second rapid test would improve the median specificity from 99.87% for the primary test to nearly 100% (95 % CI, 99.97–100) for all potential combinations. The modeling also explored the impact of population prevalence on the outcome of supplementary testing. With decreasing prevalence, the number of tests that require resolution (primary positive, secondary negative) changes little, but increasingly consists of false-positive primary tests.

Because of well-documented concerns about the specificity of oral fluid testing in some settings,[28] algorithms using oral fluid testing with two blood tests to supplement positives have been proposed. The New York City Health Department[29] implemented an algorithm in which a positive oral fluid was followed with the same rapid test on blood. Of 1194 reactive oral-fluid rapid tests that were retested, 840 of 850 (98.8%) reactive with both oral fluid and whole blood were confirmed positive. Of 344 that were negative with whole blood, 343 (99.9%) were negative by Western blot.

For testing in areas of high incidence and prevalence, the San Francisco Department of Public Health[29,30] reported strategies using an initial oral-fluid rapid test, where reactives were followed by two rapid blood tests. Of the thirty oral-fluid positive specimens, 22 were positive by the blood tests, and all of these were Western blot–positive. The 8 specimens with negative blood tests were also Western blot–negative.

Investigators from the New Jersey health department reported laboratory validation of an oral-to-blood algorithm. Serum specimens (n = 156) that screened positive on oral fluid but failed to confirm as Western blot–positive were retested by different rapid tests;[25] none were reactive, although 1 (0.6%) specimen was reactive on the same rapid test performed on blood. However, none of the samples confirmed on Western were tested with rapids. When combined with the New York and San Francisco data, this work suggests that a subsequent rapid test on whole blood can substantially improve the positive predictive value of a reactive oral-fluid test.

In general, testing schemes with a rapid screen and one or more rapid tests to confirm, as described, have lower specificity than Western blot–based approaches. Modeling of cost-effectiveness, however, suggests that a two-step rapid approach has major cost advantages over Western blot–based testing and, in resource-poor environments, this may be considered to outweigh the analytical advantage of the more complex testing.[31,32]

APPLICATIONS OF RAPID HIV TESTING
Peripartum and Prenatal Screening

Both in the United States and elsewhere, many small studies demonstrate the importance of rapid HIV testing in the perinatal period, emphasizing the value of rapid results and appropriate treatment in preventing peripartum HIV transmission.[33] In 1999, the Institute of Medicine determined that continued perinatal HIV transmission was in large part due to lack of knowledge of HIV infection status, and recommended routine prenatal HIV testing.[34] Unfortunately, women frequently present in labor with inadequate prenatal care, unaware of their serostatus, and may therefore be inadequately treated. A large multicenter clinical trial conducted by the Mother-Infant Rapid Intervention At Delivery (MIRIAD) group demonstrated that point-of-care testing is an effective approach for managing serostatus-unknown women presenting in labor. In this landmark study, rapid point-of-care HIV tests provided timely diagnosis and access to antiretroviral prophylaxis. Of the 4849 women in labor enrolled in the study, 34 were positive by the OraQuick Rapid HIV-1 Antibody Test; all were ultimately positive with conventional enzyme immunoassays and confirmatory Western blot. Eighteen of the seropositive women whose rapid HIV antibody results were available before delivery, along with all newborns born to HIV-positive women, received antiretroviral prophylaxis. Of the 32 infants with follow-up data, 3 were found to be HIV-infected. Of these 3, 2 were already DNA-positive at birth; all had been delivered vaginally, which is associated with a higher risk of infection than cesarean section. Although no control arm was employed in this study, vertical HIV transmission was rare compared with historically reported transmission rates of 25% in untreated women and infants.[35] Significantly, the testing was performed at point of care by residents and nursing staff, and the tests performed well. Overall, rapid perinatal testing shows evidence-based benefits compared with conventional HIV-testing protocols.[33]

While new technologies may improve care, often profoundly, unintended consequences are often a consequence the complex social environment in which testing occurs. In St. Petersburg, Russia, a rapid HIV-screening program was implemented in a high-prevalence labor and delivery facility, with 6.4% prevalence in unscreened mothers. The program successfully improved prophylaxis rates; the intrapartum rate rose from 41% to 76%. However, at the same time, the infant abandonment rate increased from 26% to 50%; 73% in women with unintended pregnancies.[36]

Occupational Exposure

Occupational exposure to blood and bodily fluids remains a significant risk to workers and a burden on the health care system, despite the low per-incident risk of seroconversion following these incidents. The costs and distress associated with follow-up and antiretroviral prophylaxis and treatment are significant. In many cases, these may be addressed by employing rapid point-of-care testing.[2] In 2001, using the first-generation Single Use Diagnostic System HIV-1 assay with similar performance characteristics to those currently available, the costs of treating exposed health care workers following rapid versus conventional testing of source patients was reviewed, and nearly $6000 were saved in the diagnosis and treatment of 17 exposed individuals.[37] Other studies confirmed the cost savings of rapid testing[38] and noted additional benefits, including improved source patient seroawareness and increased compliance with postexposure reporting.[39]

Outreach

No use of point-of-care HIV testing has more potential than that for outside the confines of the hospital or other health care setting. Populations that might previously have lacked access to diagnosis and treatment can be targeted. However, unless quality issues in the preanalytical, analytical, and postanalytical phases of testing are monitored and addressed, outreach testing may fall short of its potential, or even do harm.

While the quality of point-of-care HIV testing has been excellent in most settings, monitoring is essential to ensure quality is maintained, as was demonstrated by a post-marketing surveillance study of CDC-funded testing with the OraQuick at 17 city and state health departments between August 11, 2004, and June 30, 2005.[40] Overall, excellent performance was described. Tests were performed on whole blood (135,724) or oral fluid (26,066). Very high specificity was observed with whole blood (99.98%, positive predictive value [PPV] 99.24%) and oral fluid (99.89%, PPV 90.00%); 124 discordant results were reported from 68 (0.05%) whole-blood and 56 (0.22%) oral-fluid rapid tests. One site, however, reported an excess of oral-fluid false-positives. At this site, specificity was 98.7% with a PPV of 50%. Most false-positive tests were "faint" or "grey." No expired devices or unique lots were used at this site. No single operator was involved. No change in frequency was observed after a sampling discrepancy (double-swiping device instead of single-swiping) was corrected. Temperatures were within range throughout period, and no cause of the false-positive results was found; eventually oral-fluid testing was discontinued at the affected site.

Although rapid HIV tests are quite easy to use, nothing is foolproof. Performance-related errors are a concern, especially as the tests transition from a laboratory with trained technologists, to the point of care with skilled medical staff, to other outreach settings with less training and supervision, and even, potentially, to home use. A 2004 study of the OraQuick assay found increased functional error rates when the test was administered by non–laboratory workers. Result-reporting errors, transcription errors, and other clerical errors were also observed, and the investigators stated the need for ongoing training and performance assessment.[41] Other functional issues, including variability in storage, kit handling, and environmental parameters, have not been extensively studied, and may represent obstacles for point-of-care testing if users are unaware of their impact on test quality. Addressing these concerns, the CDC outlined quality-assurance and practice guidelines with recommendations to all agencies employing rapid HIV testing.[42]

The package inserts of all available rapid assays note that they are "for use only by agents of a clinical laboratory." However, the OraQuick, Uni-Gold Recombigen, and Clearview Stat-Pak are "Clinical Laboratories Improvement Amendment (CLIA) waived" for a subset of specimen types, blurring the lines of who does and does not constitute an "agent" of a clinical laboratory—and what exactly is meant by a "clinical laboratory." Concerns remain regarding the quality of testing in laboratories operating under a certificate of waiver. Such laboratories operate under minimal oversight, with extremely limited requirements for personnel or testing procedures. Alarming error rates have been observed in randomly surveyed waived-testing laboratories; training and monitoring of health care providers who administer rapid point-of-care tests are necessary to achieve the expected assay performance characteristics.[43]

Encouragingly, studies demonstrate that the barriers to outreach testing are not insurmountable. Using the OraQuick Rapid HIV-1 Antibody test, the investigators of one study demonstrated effective implementation of a straightforward screening program of high-risk homeless and marginally housed adults in San Francisco. Of the 1614 individuals approached to participate, 1213 (75.2%) underwent testing, and 187 of those were ultimately confirmed positive. All participants received counseling, testing, and referral to appropriate ancillary services, and nearly 87% reported at least one follow-up visit with a health care provider in the following months. However, of the 37 newly diagnosed cases, 7 did not return for confirmatory testing results and could not be linked to appropriate interventional services.[44]

A series of reports on the use of rapid tests in outreach settings has been summarized in an editorial to a supplemental issue of *Public Health Reports*.[45] Articles in the supplement describe real-world examples of programs designed to improve access to HIV testing by underserved groups. Testing in emergency rooms is well received by patients and may identify undiscovered cases, but may miss some groups who perceive their HIV risks as low. The use of rapid HIV tests in sexually transmitted disease clinics may improve the rate of return for sexually transmitted disease test results. In a nonclinical setting, rapid HIV tests delivered through a community-based organization detected newly infected patients who were negative when tested during the previous year and were well received by staff, but identified fewer infected persons than expected. A study of rapid HIV testing provided specifically to transgender persons reported a high rate of infection in this difficult-to-reach population. A program in historically black colleges and universities was successful in testing a substantial number of previously untested persons. Also, the use of rapid tests as part of HIV partner counseling and referral services may improve the efficiency of service and make partners more likely to be tested. Rapid HIV tests are being used in a variety of settings to detect infection earlier and, in previously underserved populations, to reach patients who most need them. However, such tests must be applied thoughtfully for optimum value.

SUMMARY

The advent, approval, distribution, and use of rapid HIV testing have changed HIV testing practices worldwide. These simple, rapid tests play diagnostic roles that were inadequately filled by conventional screening methods.[46,47] However, rapid point-of-care testing places novel demands on systems and treatment protocols to effectively address screen-positive patients. In the outreach and community settings, for example, individuals who test positive with rapid screening are still obligated to return for confirmatory testing. The impact of rapid diagnosis on behavior of patients diagnosed by point-of-care tests is still unknown. Additionally, as for conventional testing, linking HIV-positive individuals to counseling, medical, and social services and linking the high-risk HIV-negative population to prevention services are of paramount importance.[48]

All six of the approved rapid tests have good performance compared with conventional enzyme immunoassays, and fairly subtle differences with regard to other characteristics. Understanding these differences, however, may become more important as applications of rapid testing broaden.

Rapid HIV tests have become critical tools in managing the global HIV pandemic. In the setting of maternal care, particularly in the acute labor and delivery setting, they allow directed antiretroviral therapy to be given to limit perinatal spread. In the employee-health setting, they can limit the unnecessary exposure of workers to antiretroviral medications. Meanwhile, the availability of rapid, easy-to-use point-of-care HIV tests has provided new opportunities for outreach testing to reach previously untested populations in both resource-rich and resource-poor settings, detecting disease in time for early intervention to prolong life and limit the spread of HIV.

REFERENCES

1. Glynn MK, Rhodes P. Estimated HIV prevalence in the United States at the end of 2003. Presented at the 2005 National HIV Prevention Conference, Atlanta, Georgia; June 14, 2005 [abstract T1-B1101].
2. Landrum ML, Wilson CH, Perri LP, et al. Usefulness of a rapid human immunodeficiency virus-1 antibody test for the management of occupational exposure to blood and body fluid. Infect Control Hosp Epidemiol 2005;26:768–74.
3. Karon JM, Flemming PL, Steketee, et al. HIV in the United States at the turn of the century: an epidemic in transition. Am J Public Health 2001;91:1060–8.
4. Centers for Disease Control and Prevention. HIV prevention strategic plan through 2005. Atlanta (GA): CDC; 2001.
5. Holtgrave DR, Pinkerton PD. Can increasing awareness of HIV seropositivity reduce infections by 50% in the United States? J Acquir Immune defic Syndr 2007;44:360–3.
6. Marks G, Crepaz N, Janssen RS. Estimating the sexual transmission of HIV from persons aware and unaware that they are infected with the virus in the USA. AIDS 206;20:1447–50.
7. Spielberg F, Banson B, Goldbaum G, et al. Overcoming barriers to HIV testing: preferences for new strategies among clients of a needle exchange, a sexually transmitted disease clinic, and sex venues for men who have sex with men. J Acquir Immune defic Syndr 2003;32:318–27.
8. Irwin K, Olivio N, Schable CA, et al. The CDC-Bronx-Lebanon HIC Serosurvey team. Performance characteristics of a rapid HIV antibody assay in a hospital with high prevalence of HIV infection. Ann Intern Med 1996;125:471–5.

9. Spielberg F, Kassler WJ. Rapid testing for HIV antibody: a technology whose time has come. Ann Intern Med 1996;125:509–11.

10. Peterman TA, Todd KA, Mapanduki I. Opportunities of targeting publicly funded human immunodeficiency virus counseling and testing. J Acquir Immune defic Syndr 1996;12:69–74.

11. APHL/CDC. Proposed HIV test algorithms for consideration. Available at: www. hivtestingconference.org/hta.htm. Accessed April 12, 2009.

12. Campbell SM, Klein RD. Home testing for HIV—boon or bane? J Clin Microbiol 2006;44:3473–6.

13. Lee VJ, Tan SC, Earnest A, et al. User acceptability and feasibility of self-testing with HIV rapid tests. J Acquir Immune defic Syndr 2007;45(4):449–53.

14. Summary of safety and effectiveness, CBER. Oraquick Rapid HIV-1. Available at: http://www.fda.gov/cber/pmasumm/P010047S.pdf. Accessed April 10, 2007.

15. Summary of safety and effectiveness, CBER. Uni-Gold Recombigen HIV. Available at: http://www.fda.gov/cber/pmasumm/P0300250S.pdf. Accessed April 10, 2007.

16. Summary of safety and effectiveness, CBER. MedMira reveal rapid HIV-1 antibody test. Available at: http://www.fda.gov/cber/pmasumm/P000023S.htm. Accessed April 10, 2007.

17. Summary of safety and effectiveness, CBER. Bio-rad multispot HIV-1/HIV-2 rapid test. Available at: http://www.fda.gov/cber/pmasumm/P040046S.pdf. Accessed April 10, 2007.

18. Summary of safety and effectiveness, CBER. Chembio HIV 1/2 STAT-PAK assay. Available at: http://www.fda.gov/cber/pmasumm/P050010S.pdf. Accessed April 10, 2007.

19. O'Connell RJ, Merritt TM, Malia JA, et al. Perfomance of the OraQuick rapid antibody test in diagnosis of human immunodeficiency virus type 1 infection in patients with various levels of exposure to highly active antiretroviral therapy. J Clin Microbiol 2003;41:2153–5.

20. Louie B, Wong E, Klausner JD, et al. Assessment of rapid tests for detection of human immunodeficiency virus–specific antibodies in recently infected individuals. J Clin Microbiol 2008;46:1494–7.

21. Menard D, Mairo A, Mandeng MJ, et al. Evaluation of rapid HIV testing strategies in under equipped laboratories in the Central African Republic. J Virol Methods 2005;126:75–80.

22. Menard D, Mavolomade EE, Mandeng MJ, et al. Advantages of an alternative strategy based on consecutive HIV serological tests for detection of HIV antibodies in Central African Republic. J Virol Methods 2003;111:129–34.

23. Urassa W, Nozohoor S, Jaffer S, et al. Evaluation of an alternative confirmatory strategy for the diagnosis of HIV infection in Dar Es Salaam, Tanzania, based on simple rapid assays. J Virol Methods 2002;100:115–20.

24. Boromisa R. Evaluation of a 3 rapid test algorithm for the diagnosis of HIV infection at point of care rapid testing facilities: strategy 4 data needs. 2007 HIV Diagnostics Conference, oral presentation. Available at: http://www.hivtestingconference.org/powerpoint/4_Boromisa.pps. Accessed April 12, 2009.

25. Cadoff E. Retrospective application of the proposed CDC/APHL rapid testing algorithm in New Jersey 2004–2007. 2007 HIV Diagnostics Conference, oral presentation. Available at: http://www.hivtestingconference.org/powerpoint/2_Cadoff.pps. Accessed April 12, 2009.

26. Haukoos J. Implementing a laboratory-based rapid HIV testing algorithm using two different test kits in a hospital emergency department. 2007 HIV Diagnostics

Conference, oral presentation. Available at: http://www.hivtestingconference.org/powerpoint/3_Boyett.pps. Accessed April 12, 2009.

27. Delaney K. Comparing the performance of the APHL/CDC proposed POC testing strategies and other potential options using data from the CDC's evaluation of FDA approved rapid tests. 2007 HIV Diagnostics Conference, oral presentation. Available at: http://www.hivtestingconference.org/powerpoint/3_Delaney.pps 2007. Accessed April 12, 2009.

28. Centers for Disease Control and Prevention. False-positive oral fluid rapid HIV tests—New York City, 2005–2008. MMWR Morb Mortal Wkly Rep 57:660–5.

29. Knoble T. Implementing a multiple rapid HIV test algorithm to quickly identify false positive rapid tests and provide immediate referral to care for persons likely to be infected with HIV, San Francisco, CA 2007. 2007 HIV Diagnostic Conference, oral presentation. Available at: http://www.hivtestingconference.org/powerpoint/4_Knoble.pps. Accessed April 12, 2009.

30. Dowling T. Training and quality assurance for a rapid test algorithm: lessons from implementation, San Francisco, CA 2007. 2007 HIV Diagnostic Conference, oral presentation. Available at: http://www.hivtestingconference.org/powerpoint/2_Dowling.pps. Accessed April 12, 2009.

31. Wright RJ, Stringer JS. Rapid testing strategies for HIV-1 serodiagnosis in high-prevalence African settings. Am J Prev Med 2004;27:42–8.

32. Ekwueme DU, Pinkerton SD, Holtgrave DR, et al. Cost comparison of three HIV counseling and testing technologies. Am J Prev Med 2003;25:112–21.

33. Pai NP, Tulsky JP, Cohan D, et al. Rapid point-of-care HIV testing in pregnant women: a systematic review and meta-analysis. Trop Med Int Health 2007; 12(2):162–73.

34. Institute of Medicine, National Research Council. Reducing the odds: preventing perinatal transmission of HIV in the United States. Washington, DC: National Academy Press; 1999.

35. Bulterys M, Jamieson DJ, O'Sullivan MJ, et al. Mother-Infant Rapid Intervention at Delivery (MIRIAD) Study Group. Rapid HIV-1 testing during labour: a multicenter study. JAMA 2004;292:219–23.

36. Hillis SD, Rakhmanova A, Vinogradova E, et al. Rapid HIV testing, pregnancy, antiretroviral prophylaxis and infant abandonment in St. Petersburg. Int J STD AIDS 2007;18:120–2.

37. Kallenborn JC, Price TG, Carrico RC, et al. Emergency department management of occupational exposures: cost analysis of rapid HIV test. Infect Control Hosp Epidemiol 2001;22:289–93.

38. Machado AA, Martinez R, Haikal AA, et al. Advantages of the rapid HIV-1 test in occupational accidents with potentially contaminated material among health workers. Rev Inst Med Trop Sao Paulo 2001;43:199–201.

39. Puro V, Fraincisci D, Sighinolfi L, et al. Benefits of a rapid HIV test for evaluation of the source patient after occupational exposure of healthcare workers. J Hosp Infect 2004;57:179–82.

40. Wesolowski LG, MacKellar DA, Facente SN, et al. Post-marketing surveillance of OraQuick whole blood and oral fluid rapid HIV testing. CDC, HIV/AIDS surveillance report. Atlanta (GA): US Department of Health and Human Services; 2006. 2005:1-5320:1661–6.

41. Granade TC, Parekh BS, Phillips SK, et al. Performance of he OraQuick and Hema-strip rapid HIV antibody detection assays by non-laboratorians. J Clin Virol 2004;30:229–32.

42. CDC. Quality assurance guidelines for testing using the OraQuick rapid HIV-1 antibody test. Atlanta (GA): US Department of Health and Human Services; 2003.

43. CDC. Good laboratory practices for waived testing sites survey findings from testing sites holding a certificate of waiver under the clinical laboratory improvement amendments of 1988 and recommendations for promoting quality testing. MMWR Morb Mortal Wkly Rep 2005;54(RR-13):1–25.

44. Bucher JB, Thomas KM, Guzman D, et al. Community-based rapid HIV testing in homeless and marginally housed adults in San Francisco. HIV Med 2007;8: 28–31.

45. Sanchez TH, Sullivan PS. Expanding the horizons: new approaches to providing HIV testing services in the United States. Public Health Rep 2008;123(Suppl 3): 1–4.

46. Campbell S, Campos J, Hall GS, et al. Chapter 8. Infectious diseases. In: National Academy of Clinical Biochemistry laboratory medicine practice guidelines: evidence-based practice for point-of-care testing, Nichols J, editor. 2007.

47. Galvan FH, Books RA, Leibowitz AA. Rapid HIV testing: issues in implementation. AIDS Patient Care STDs 2004;18:15–8.

48. UNAIDS, WHO, UNICEF. Towards universal access: scaling up priority HIV/AIDS interventions in the health sector. Progress report April 2007. Available at: http://www.who.int/hiv/mediacentre/universal_access_progress_report_en.pdf. Accessed April 12, 2009.

Drug-of-Abuse Testing at the Point of Care

Stacy E.F. Melanson, MD, PhD

KEYWORDS

• Drugs of abuse • Point-of-care • Substance abuse
• Clinical laboratory • Emergency department
• Pain management

Sensitive and specific assays are available to detect drugs of abuse at the point of care. This article describes the characteristics of point-of-care devices for drug-of-abuse testing with a focus on clinical utility and patient care. This article is not a comprehensive review of all available point-of-care devices. Instead it discusses general principles of point-of-care testing for drugs of abuse.

CLINICAL UTILITY

Substance abuse is a significant problem in the United States. For this reason, drug-of-abuse testing is administered in a variety of settings and includes testing for substances commonly misused recreationally, such as opiates, cocaine, amphetamines, cannabinoids, and benzodiazepines. As many as 50% of emergency-room visits are related to drug or alcohol use and clinicians rely on accurate test results to assess and manage these patients.[1,2] Drug-of-abuse testing is also frequently employed in pain-management centers to assess compliance and detect use of undisclosed or illicit substances.[3,4]

Because results can be obtained so quickly, point-of-care testing for drugs of abuse may be preferable in many clinical settings, such as emergency departments, drug treatment clinics, and detoxification clinics, and in settings related to maternal fetal medicine and pain management. A study done in the emergency department of a large academic hospital showed that point-of-care drug-of-abuse testing decreased length of stay and result turnaround time.[5] Point-of-care testing also allows clinicians to more effectively manage patients by taking clinical action immediately.

Several manufacturers have developed drug-of-abuse assays that offer similar sensitivity and specificity to the methodologies used by central laboratories. For such assays, assay performance is acceptable. However, point-of-care testing has disadvantages compared to central laboratory testing, including a less comprehensive test menu. Result interpretation may also be subjective, making performance

Division of Clinical Laboratories, Department of Pathology, Brigham and Women's Hospital, 75 Francis Street, Amory 2-217F, Boston, MA 02115, USA
E-mail address: semelanson@partners.org

Clin Lab Med 29 (2009) 503–509
doi:10.1016/j.cll.2009.06.010
0272-2712/09/$ – see front matter © 2009 Elsevier Inc. All rights reserved.

operator-dependent. Furthermore, proper documentation of results in the patients record can be problematic. Higher cost and accuracy of billing should also be considered when implementing drug-of-abuse testing at the point of care.[6–8]

POINT-OF-CARE DEVICES

A number of point-of-care devices are available to screen for drugs of abuse. These include Triage Drugs of Abuse Panels and Triage TOX Drug Screens (Biosite, Inc., San Diego, California), OnTrak TesTcard 9 (Varian, Inc., Palo Alto, California), Rapid Drug Screen (American Bio Medica, Kinderhook, New York), Intercept (OraSure Technologies, Inc., Bethlehem, Pennsylvania), Profile-II (MEDTOX Diagnostics, Burlington, North Carolina), and Status DS (LifeSign LLC, Somerset, New Jersey).[9] A solid-phase immunoassay with a visible end point in a disposable cartridge is usually employed where the target analyte migrates along a chromogenic strip and competes with antibody at a specified location with resultant loss or formation of a colored line. Device formats include dipsticks, cup devices, cards, and plastic cassettes. Some devices can be performed in one step after depositing the sample in the collection container. Other devices require pipetting and incubation steps.

In recent years, a number of drug-of-abuse devices for self-testing in the home have become available over-the-counter at shopping malls and drug stores. One is First Check (Selection Management, Woodland, Texas). Some over-the-counter devices use a urine sample to test for a single drug, while others test for a panel of drugs. One manufacturer markets a device for collection of a hair sample that is subsequently sent to a laboratory. These new devices reflect a perceived need by some members of the public to have access to drug-of-abuse testing outside of the traditional medical establishment for either testing of family members or testing of themselves to ensure satisfactory results prior to providing an employment or drug-rehabilitation specimen. One major advantage, other than convenience, is that home testing generates no record of the results, ensuring patient privacy. However, the social consequences of a false-positive result when a family member is tested needs consideration.

SPECIMEN TYPES

Urine is the specimen of choice for most of the devices and the window of detection in urine for most drugs of abuse, with the exception of cannabinoids, is approximately 2 to 3 days.[1] Required volumes vary from a few drops to 30 mL, depending on the device. One consideration for urine testing is that visually turbid urine or urine containing sediment may require precentrifugation to avoid false-negative results.[8] In addition, clinicians must be aware of adulteration techniques and preanalytical variables, such as those involving pH, specific gravity, aroma, and appearance, that can be used to detect adulterants.[1]

Due to the difficulty and inconvenience of urine collection, as well as the possibility of adulteration, the use of alternative samples for drug-of-abuse testing has been explored.[6,8,10] Oral fluid (saliva) is easy to collect, noninvasive, and unlikely to be adulterated. Saliva testing avoids the need to observe patients providing a urine specimen. This is particularly important if an observer of the appropriate gender is not available to witness the urine collection. The parent drugs, not the metabolites, are present in saliva and the window of detection is different than that for urine. For this reason, drugs may be detectable earlier in saliva than in urine. Thus, results from saliva may be more reflective of current impairment. The Intercept device screens for drugs of abuse in saliva. The panel includes cannabinoids, cocaine, opiates, phencyclidine, amphetamines, methamphetamine (including ecstasy), benzodiazepines, and methadone. By accommodating saliva testing, OraSure offers an advantage in some situations where an acceptable urine specimen cannot be reliably collected.

Saliva-based testing has several disadvantages. Screening for drugs in saliva can be analytically challenging because analytes are present in lower concentrations and the sample volumes are smaller. For example, oral fluid is a poor specimen for cannabinoid detection.[1] Oral contamination and pH effects can influence test results in saliva, so preanalytical variables should be carefully considered. In some cases, patients abusing stimulants, such as amphetamine or ecstasy, may not be able to provide an adequate specimen. Finally, there is little information concerning interferences seen with saliva-based testing.

Other specimen types for drug-of-abuse testing include sweat, hair, nail, and meconium. Sweat collection is impractical. Elimination through the skin may be delayed for many days, collection is prone to external contamination, and concentrations may differ depending on the collection site. Hair, nail, and meconium are not suitable for point of care because extraction procedures are required to isolate the drugs. Breath alcohol devices are also available with primary use for law enforcement outside clinical settings.[8,11]

TEST MENU

Although the test menu for each manufacturer differs, most platforms screen for drugs included in the National Institute of Drug Abuse (NIDA) 5 panel (amphetamine, opiates, cannabinoids, phencyclidine, and cocaine). The NIDA 5 drugs do not typically satisfy the requirements in hospital settings. For example, the emergency department, to assess and adequately manage overdose situations, requires tricyclic antidepressants, barbiturates, acetaminophen, salicyclate, and ethanol. The lack of point-of-care devices that perform the basic panel required by the emergency department reflects the emphasis by manufacturers on medicolegal drug-of-abuse testing rather than on clinical toxicology performed mainly to aid in the medical management of the patient. Because of the limitations in the test menu, many hospitals have not implemented drug-of-abuse testing at the point of care. Several different panels offer configurations that include amphetamines, methamphetamines, barbiturates, benzodiazepines, cocaine, methadone, opiates, phencyclidine, propoxyphene, tricyclic antidepressants, cannabinoids, and acetaminophen.[9] Only salicylate and ethanol are missing, although ethanol is often measured by breathalyzer or other means.

Demand has increased for drug-of-abuse testing in pain-management centers to determine compliance with chronic opioid therapy and detect use of undisclosed or illicit substances. Point-of-care devices offer the advantage of immediate counseling for unsuspected results and timely prescription renewal for suspected results. In part to accommodate point-of-care testing in pain clinics, the range of available point-of-care tests has expanded to include buprenorphine, oxycodone, and the methadone metabolite 2-ethylidene-1,5-dimethyl-3,3-diphenylpyrrolidine (EDDP).[12,13]

METHODOLOGY

Most point-of-care devices for drug-of-abuse testing are immunoassays, which employ agglutination reactions, chromogenic antibodies, chromogenic drug conjugates, fluorescent antibody conjugates, or fluorescent drug conjugates. Depending on the assay, antibodies are designed to detect a specific drug of abuse (eg, methadone), a metabolite (eg, benzoylecgonine), or a class of compounds (eg, opiates). Qualitative results are based on a specific calibrator concentration. Positive results reflect a concentration above the calibrator cutoff, while negative results reflect concentrations below the cutoff and do not exclude the presence of a drug or its metabolite.

Most devices are competitive immunoassays in which the absence of a line indicates the presence of a specific drug or class of drug. This configuration is somewhat counterintuitive because most point-of-care tests use the appearance of a line as the indication of a positive test. A drug conjugate is impregnated on a membrane and a free antibody is coated on microparticles. If sufficient drug is present in the patient's urine, the drug binds to the free antibody, the free antibody is subsequently inhibited from binding to the drug conjugate on the membrane, and no band is formed. However, assays are available in which a positive response indicates the presence of the drug.

The complexity and length of the assays vary. One device requires three steps and two timed periods, which increases the complexity of the assay as well as the turn-around time.[8,9,14] Typically, results can be obtained in less than 15 minutes. However, some devices require 15 to 30 minutes.[15,16]

ANALYTICAL PERFORMANCE

The analytical performance, including sensitivity, specificity, precision, and accuracy of point-of-care drug-of-abuse devices have been addressed in several studies.[9,14–23] Most studies suggest that point-of-care testing is a reliable method to screen for drugs of abuse and that results are comparable to both those from automated immunoassays and those from the gold standard, gas chromatography/mass spectrometry (GC/MS). However, a few inconsistencies have been noted by studies examining each of these devices. Taylor and colleagues[24] found that several products, including the American Bio Medica Rapid Drug Screen and the LifeSign Status DS, have discrepancies between manufacturer claims and product performance. In addition, some devices do not adhere to their stated cutoffs and show positive results below the cutoff and negative results above the cutoff.[9] In one study, the Triage gave positive results below the cannabinoids and cocaine metabolite cutoffs and negative results above the amphetamine cutoff.[14] These inconsistencies are not unexpected and, for clinical purposes, minor differences in performance at the cutoff are not likely to be clinically important. However, the laboratory should inform clinicians that immunoassays for drugs of abuse, whether performed at the point of care or in the laboratory, are qualitative screening tests and all results should be confirmed using a definitive technique such as GC/MS.

Cross-reactivity differs among point-of-care devices because of the differences in antibody specificity. The antibody specificity varies within the drug class and each individual drug within the class requires a different urine concentration to trigger a positive result. In addition, antibodies may be designed to cross-react with the metabolite to allow for longer detection window, which changes the cross-reactivity profile to the parent compound. Certain antibodies may also cross-react with medications outside the target class, leading to false-positive results.

The manufacturer should provide a list of compounds tested and their degree of cross-reactivity, including those medications outside the drug class, which may cause false-positive results. Cyclobenzaprine may cross-react in the tricyclic assay and pantoprazole may trigger a positive result with the cannabinoid assay. Diphenhydramine and tricyclic antidepressants may cross-react in the propoxyphene assay, but at concentrations significantly above the pharmacologic range.[19] Virtually all drug-of-abuse test systems, because their methodology is immunoassay, exhibit false-positive results and cross-react outside the drug or drug class. For this reason, the laboratory and clinicians must be familiar with the idiosyncrasies of the specific device employed at the point of care.

RESULT INTERPRETATION AND DOCUMENTATION

Result interpretation and result documentation are important for accurate accessible results, especially at the point of care. Unlike automated platforms, most steps are operator-dependent, including sample application, timing of reaction, and interpretation of a visual end point. With most point-of-care drug-of-abuse devices, the absence of a line indicates that a drug is present at or above the defined threshold and even a faint line should be interpreted as negative. Furthermore, the window to read the result is typically 5 to 10 minutes and, if an operator extends the read time, false results can be obtained. The Triage TOX Drug Screens offer the advantage of a one-step method and an instrument-read cartridge that avoids the need to visually interpret multiple bands and permits results to be interfaced directly to the laboratory information system. The accuracy and reliability of point-of-care testing for drugs of abuse may be improved by providing interpretative comments to illustrate differences in sensitivity and specificity and facilitate interpretation.

REGULATORY COMPLIANCE

Departments considering the implementation of point-of-care devices should collaborate with the laboratory on several levels, including device selection, assay validation, training and competency, device usage audits, result reporting, and laboratory information system interfaces. Collaboration is particularly important for drug-of-abuse testing because of the potential for false-negative and false-positive results.

Point-of-care testing is complicated by the frequent involvement of nonlaboratory personnel in quality control, interpretation, and documentation. Tests must be simple and easy to perform with unambiguous interpretation so no false-negative or false-positive results are obtained as the result of unskilled personnel. Devices should be evaluated and validated under typical working conditions to assess the effects from many variables, such as distractions from multitasking workers and improper lighting. Quality-control and quality-assurance procedures, which are routine in the clinical laboratory, may be less familiar to those performing point-of-care testing. Internal controls are used to indicate insufficient sample or improper migration. Additional external controls may also be necessary with new reagent lots or new instrument operators.

Even if all of the testing steps are performed properly, documentation of results in the patient's medical record can be problematic. Some devices offer the added benefit of quality-control lockouts, programmable quality-control intervals, printed reports, and the ability to interface to the laboratory information system, thus ensuring that testing performed by nonlaboratory personnel is compliant with quality-control and documentation requirements.

Point-of-care testing is a rapid and accurate way to screen for drugs of abuse. When evaluating or choosing a point-of-care device, certain features should be considered, such as clinical utility, reliability of device manufacturer, specimen type, test menu, methodology, analytical performance, regulatory compliance, result interpretation and documentation, and cost.

REFERENCES

1. Watson I. Clinical drug testing at the point of care. 2nd edition. Washington (DC): AACC Press; 2004.
2. Wu AH, McKay C, Broussard LA, et al. National academy of clinical biochemistry laboratory medicine practice guidelines: recommendations for the use of

laboratory tests to support poisoned patients who present to the emergency department. Clin Chem 2003;49(3):357–79.

3. Heit HA, Gourlay DL. Urine drug testing in pain medicine. J Pain Symptom Manage 2004;27(3):260–7.

4. Trescot AM, Boswell MV, Atluri SL, et al. Opioid guidelines in the management of chronic non-cancer pain. Pain Physician 2006;9(1):1–39.

5. Lewandrowski K, Flood J, Finn C, et al. Implementation of point-of-care rapid urine testing for drugs of abuse in the emergency department of an academic medical center: impact on test utilization and ED length of stay. Am J Clin Pathol 2008;129(5):796–801.

6. George S, Braithwaite RA. Use of on-site testing for drugs of abuse. Clin Chem 2002;48(10):1639–46.

7. Hicks JM, Haeckel R, Price CP, et al. Recommendations and opinions for the use of point-of-care testing for hospitals and primary care: summary of a 1999 symposium. Clin Chim Acta 2001;303(1–2):1–17.

8. Watson I, Bertholf R, Hammett-Stabler C, et al. Drugs and ethanol. Washington (DC): National Academy of Clinical Biochemistry; 2006.

9. Leino A, Saarimies J, Gronholm M, et al. Comparison of eight commercial on-site screening devices for drugs-of-abuse testing. Scand J Clin Lab Invest 2001; 61(4):325–31.

10. Pil K, Verstraete A. Current developments in drug testing in oral fluid. Ther Drug Monit 2008;30(2):196–202.

11. Bendtsen P, Hultberg J, Carlsson M, et al. Monitoring ethanol exposure in a clinical setting by analysis of blood, breath, saliva, and urine. Alcohol Clin Exp Res 1999;23(9):1446–51.

12. Haller CA, Stone J, Burke V, et al. Comparison of an automated and point-of-care immunoassay to GC-MS for urine oxycodone testing in the clinical laboratory. J Anal Toxicol 2006;30(2):106–11.

13. Leino A, Loo BM. Comparison of three commercial tests for buprenorphine screening in urine. Ann Clin Biochem 2007;44(Pt 6):563–5.

14. Phillips JE, Bogema S, Fu P, et al. Signify ER Drug Screen Test evaluation: comparison to Triage Drug of Abuse Panel plus tricyclic antidepressants. Clin Chim Acta 2003;328(1–2):31–8.

15. Schwartz JG, Hurd IL, Carnahan JJ. Determination of tricyclic antidepressants for ED analysis. Am J Emerg Med 1994;12(5):513–6.

16. Yang JM, Lewandrowski KB. Urine drugs of abuse testing at the point-of-care: clinical interpretation and programmatic considerations with specific reference to the Syva Rapid Test (SRT). Clin Chim Acta 2001;307(1–2):27–32.

17. de la Torre R, Domingo-Salvany A, Badia R, et al. Clinical evaluation of the Triage analytic device for drugs-of-abuse testing. Clin Chem 1996;42(9):1433–8.

18. Mastrovitch TA, Bithoney WG, DeBari VA, et al. Point-of-care testing for drugs of abuse in an urban emergency department. Ann Clin Lab Sci 2002;32(4):383–6.

19. Poklis A, Poklis JL, Tarnai LD, et al. Evaluation of the Triage PPY on-site testing device for the detection of dextropropoxyphene in urine. J Anal Toxicol 2004; 28(6):485–8.

20. Taylor EH, Pizzo P. Evaluation of the DrugCheck 9 on-site immunoassay test cup according to a standard method validation protocol. J Anal Toxicol 2004;28(3): 190–7.

21. Moody DE, Fang WB, Andrenyak DM, et al. A comparative evaluation of the instant-view 5-panel test card with OnTrak TesTcup Pro 5: comparison with gas chromatography-mass spectrometry. J Anal Toxicol 2006;30(1):50–6.

22. Tomaszewski C, Runge J, Gibbs M, et al. Evaluation of a rapid bedside toxicology screen in patients suspected of drug toxicity. J Emerg Med 2005;28(4):389–94.

23. Wu AH, Wong SS, Johnson KG, et al. Evaluation of the triage system for emergency drugs-of-abuse testing in urine. J Anal Toxicol 1993;17(4):241–5.

24. Taylor EH, Oertli EH, Wolfgang JW, et al. Accuracy of five on-site immunoassay drugs-of-abuse testing devices. J Anal Toxicol 1999;23(2):119–24.

Tight Glycemic Control and Point-of-Care Testing

David Alter, MD[a],*, Greg Deines, DO[b]

> **KEYWORDS**
> - Tight glycemic control • Point-of-care testing • Glucometer
> - Blood glucose • Hyperglycemia

According to the hypothesis of tight glycemic control (TGC), inpatient morbidity and mortality will be reduced by processes and practices that "tightly" maintain blood glucose levels within a strictly defined range regardless of diabetic status (diabetes or not), acuity of illness, or admitting diagnosis. Until 2001, inpatient glycemic management focused solely on the diabetic patient with few reported studies that discussed hyperglycemic management of the nondiabetic patient. However, scattered studies looked at the prognostic impact of hyperglycemia in the nondiabetic inpatient population. One such study from 1975 dealt with the prognostic impact of hyperglycemia in the post–myocardial infarction population.[1] This study noted that patients with higher fasting blood-glucose levels within 72 hours of admission had a higher mortality.

For the last 35 years, the prevailing notion was that hyperglycemia in the acutely ill nondiabetic inpatient was a consequence of illnesses as well as a marker of its severity. Hyperglycemia was also thought to be an adaptive response to injury necessary for survival and not necessarily a prognostic indicator of morbidity or mortality.[2,3] In this article, we discuss the current school of thought regarding prognostic implications of nondiabetic inpatient hyperglycemia, its management to achieve TGC, and the relationship of point-of-care testing to TGC.

Inpatient hyperglycemia is referred to as *stress hyperglycemia* and has both endogenous and exogenous metabolic pathways. Endogenously, acute illness triggers insulin resistance (in 80% of critical-care patients), as well as a release of hormones associated with elevated blood-glucose levels, such as glucagon, epinephrine, cortisol, and growth hormone.[3] Exogenously, hyperglycemia results from the use of total parenteral nutrition and dextrose infusions.[4]

---

[a] Department of Pathology and Laboratory Medicine, Spectrum Health, 1840 Wealthy St., Grand Rapids, MI 49506, USA
[b] Center for Diabetes and Endocrinology, Michigan Medical, P.C., 4069 Lake Drive SE, Suite 315, Grand Rapids, MI 49546, USA
* Corresponding author.
E-mail address: david.alter@spectrum-health.org (D. Alter).

Clin Lab Med 29 (2009) 511–522
doi:10.1016/j.cll.2009.06.009
labmed.theclinics.com

For the diabetic inpatient, strict glycemic control is quality patient standard of care, especially in light of the Diabetes Control and Complications Trial, a prospective randomized trial that extended more than 6 years and followed outpatient insulin-dependent diabetics with minimal or no diabetic complications split into intensive and routine treatment groups.[5] The results of the Diabetes Control and Complications Trial, published in 1993, demonstrated that TGC in the outpatient, as evidenced by hemoglobin A1c values, "effectively delays the onset and slows the progression of diabetic retinopathy, nephropathy and neuropathy in patients with insulin-dependent diabetes mellitus." The agreed-upon current recommendations for outpatient glycemic control[6–8] depend on a measure of the individual's glycemic status. In this group of individuals (diabetic outpatients), blood-glucose levels are obtained via self-monitoring of blood glucose using whole-blood capillary (finger-stick) specimens and every third to fourth month assays of glycated hemoglobin.

Elevated blood glucose is not a benign condition. On a cellular level, high blood-glucose levels impair neutrophil function with a subsequent overall impact on the immune system.[9] It is hypothesized that healthy cells protect against glycemic toxicity by the down-regulation of glucose transporters (GLUT-1, GLUT-2, and GLUT-3), while acute cytokines angiotensin II, endothelin-1, vascular endothelial growth factor, transforming growth factor beta, and hypoxia cause an up-regulation of those transporters, resulting in a overall influx of glucose. Excessive transport of glucose into the cell causes an increase in mitochondrial superoxide production and subsequent reactive species that directly affect normal protein structure and function.[9,10] Hyperglycemia has also been associated with a prothrombotic effect, higher free fatty acid concentrations (linked to increased risk for arrhythmias), and impaired use of myocardial glucose.[11] However, despite the increasing scientific evidence of cellular function impairment, hyperglycemia in nondiabetic patients has been of little concern because of its transient (limited to the course of the acute illness) nature. This changed in 2001.

A paradigm shift toward the management of stress hyperglycemia followed a landmark study published in November 2001[12] and several subsequent studies that demonstrated improved patient outcomes with TGC in the intensive care (surgical intensive care unit [SICU] and medical intensive care unit [MICU]) population using insulin regimens that kept blood-glucose levels in predetermined ranges. Van den Berghe and her colleagues studied 1548 SICU patients (most of these patients were postoperative; the exact percentage of non-postoperative cases was not given) on mechanical ventilation over a period of 1 year with patients randomly assigned to either intensive (n = 765, intravenous insulin to maintain glucose between 80 and 110 mg/dL) or conventional (n = 783, intravenous insulin to maintain glucose between 180 and 200 mg/dL) insulin therapy. Both groups had a similar percentage of known diabetics (13%) with similar percentages of patients treated with insulin (4% in conventional and 5% in intensive). The study demonstrated marked improvements in care in the intensive insulin therapy group. Intensive care unit (ICU) mortality was reduced by 32% (P<.04) with 35 deaths in the intensive group versus 63 deaths in the conventional group. Intensive treatment reduced ICU, but not total hospital, length of stay. In addition, fewer patients in the intensive group required prolonged ventilatory support or renal replacement therapy. Fewer episodes of septicemia and lower use of antibiotics were also seen in the intensive group.

Van den Berghe's group[13] published a follow-up study in 2006 that complemented the initial one. In this study, investigators studied hyperglycemia and outcomes in an MICU where the three primary reasons for study exclusion were ICU length of stay less than 3 days, do not resuscitate order on admission, or postoperative patient. Twelve hundred patients were identified and similarly randomized to conventional or intensive insulin protocols. Of the initial 1200, approximately 380 in each group stayed in the MICU for longer than 3 days. The results of this study were not as conclusive as the initial one. Overall, mortality did not differ between the two groups. However, for those patients with an MICU length of stay greater than 3 days, mortality was reduced from 52.5% to 43% ($P = .009$). A similar reduction in mortality was also seen for those patients with an MICU length of stay greater than 5 days. In terms of morbidity, the intensive insulin group did have a significant difference secondary to a reduction in newly acquired kidney injury (8.95 versus 5.9%, $P = .04$). In addition studies to involving the ICU population, TGC has also been studied for other conditions, two of which are acute myocardial infarction and cardiac surgery.

Hyperglycemia and its impact on the prognosis of acute myocardial infarction have also been studied at least since 1975.[1] In the last 15 years, additional studies have dealt with the impact of hyperglycemia on post–acute myocardial infarction prognosis.[14] The overall conclusion of these studies is that admission glucose and mortality are positively associated regardless of patient diabetic status; however, the risk is higher in the nondiabetic population.[15] Despite inconsistent evidence to support intensive glycemic control in the acute myocardial infarction population, TGC is recommended, as confirmed in the 2008 American Heart Association Scientific statement "Hyperglycemia and Acute Coronary Syndrome."[11] The statement clearly addresses the limited evidence for a causal relationship between hyperglycemia and adverse outcome and the lack of available consensus standards of care. The guideline says there is "currently insufficient evidence to consider glucose control as a quality measure during ACS [acute coronary syndrome] hospitalization" yet supports maintenance of glucose levels below 180 mg/dL in all patients admitted with ACS and advocates the use of insulin as the most effective method to ensure such maintenance.

The Society of Thoracic Surgeons has recently published practice guidelines on blood-glucose management during adult cardiac surgery.[16] Its key points are paraphrased below:

> Good perioperative glycemic control is necessary to prevent increased morbidity and mortality in both diabetic and nondiabetic patients.
>
> Though a glucose cutoff has not been clearly determined, less than 180 mg/dL is recommended for all patients, with insulin use suggested for diabetic patients and "as needed" for nondiabetic patients.
>
> These recommendations for glycemic control are extended to all patients postoperatively in all unit types (ICU, step-down, and floor units).

Multiple studies have followed the original Van den Berghe study and there has not been total agreement as to the original outcomes. A 2008 meta-analysis published in the *Journal of the American Medical Association* discusses this topic in some detail.[17] It identified 1358 studies of tight versus usual glucose control in the intensive care population. Twenty-nine randomized trials (8432 patients) from these studies met inclusion criteria for the analysis. The investigators concluded that tight glucose control "was not associated with a significant reduction in hospital mortality or in new need for dialysis." The study did show a significant overall reduction in septicemia with the most pronounced reduction in the SICU population. However, the study did show a fivefold increase in the rate of hypoglycemia in institutions that used TGC. The investigators also concluded that, based on evidence showing no change in mortality and increased risk of hypoglycemia with TGC, implementation of guidelines "in all critically ill patients should be reevaluated until the results of larger, more definitive clinical trials are available."

The accompanying editorial[18] tempers the conclusion of the meta-analysis by pointing out that it illustrated several global issues with studying the effects of TGC, such as inconsistency in achievement of glycemic goals throughout the studies and no standard for reporting of glycemic control (mean morning blood glucose versus percent time within target range versus time spent in hyperglycemic range versus absolute concentration and/or degree of variability). In addition, as will be discussed, there appears to be no consistency of specimen type and assay methodology used to generate a blood-glucose result.[19]

The results of the NICE-SUGAR (Normoglycemia in Intensive Care Evaluation—Survival Using Glucose Algorithm Regulation)[20] trial were published in the March 26, 2009, issue of *The New England Journal of Medicine*. NICE-SUGAR is a multicenter trial from Australia, New Zealand, and Canada that randomly assigned ICU (medical and surgical) patients to one of two groups, one where the blood-glucose level was kept at 81 to 108 mg/dL (intensive, n = 3050) and the other at less than 180 mg/dL (conventional, n = 3054) using insulin as needed to maintain those ranges. Investigators noted that, in the intensive group, severe hypoglycemia was more frequent (6.8% versus 0.5%, $P < .001$) and mortality higher (27.5% versus 24. 9%).

The study's conclusion stated: "…we do not recommend use of the lower target in critically ill adults." As a result, the medical community now faces the possibility that intensive glycemic control can actually increase mortality. The reader is referred to the accompanying editorial for a review of the issues and discussion of the unanswered questions.[21] In short, the editorial's position was that TGC has institutionalized itself around the world and abandonment of current practices would potentially do more harm than good. The solution might be to maintain blood-glucose levels less rigidly than has been proposed.

In May of 2009, the American Association of Clinical Endocrinologists and American Diabetic Association released a consensus statement on inpatient glycemic control.[22] This document is the best review of the subject and the reader is strongly recommended to review its contents. The consensus panel focused on eight questions:

Does improving glycemic control improve clinical outcomes for inpatients with hyperglycemia?
What glycemic targets can be recommended in different patient populations?
What treatment options are available for achieving optimal glycemic targets safely and effectively in specific clinical situations?
Does inpatient management of hyperglycemia represent a safety concern?
What systems need to be in place to achieve these recommendations?
Is treatment of inpatient hyperglycemia cost-effective?
What are the optimal strategies for transition to outpatient care?
What are areas for future research?

Two of most important conclusions are: (1) Some form of glycemic control for all inpatients is warranted; and (2) blood-glucose levels less stringent than 80 to 110 mg/dL with a range of 140 to 180 mg/dL are recommended.

The evidence is strong that hyperglycemia impairs neutrophil function and predisposes to infection and possibly sepsis. In addition, a consistent reduction in septicemia has been identified. Furthermore, multiple medical specialties have published recent recommendations for glycemic management giving cutoffs at less than 180 mg/dL.[11,15,16] As a result, TGC as a required practice is now approaching a standard of care in the hospital community secondary to all to the literature being generated on the subject. This has not gone unnoticed by the Centers for Medicare and Medicaid Services, which has started discussions to include poor glycemic control (both hyperglycemia and hypoglycemia) as a hospital-acquired condition, which would mean that hospitals would not be reimbursed when complications related to poor glycemic control occur during an inpatient stay.[23]

Unfortunately, there is a lot of debate as to what constitutes hyperglycemia and over such questions as: What's causing the benefit (insulin itself, decreased blood glucose, or combination of both)? and Is the risk of hypoglycemic sequelae worth the benefit of better glycemic control? TGC hinges on the blood-glucose result, with the expectation that it is as accurate and precise as possible. Since TGC processes require a rapid blood-glucose result for real-time insulin-drip adjustment, the necessity of point-of-care glucose testing rises to the forefront.

The cornerstone of TGC is a blood-glucose result with a rapid turnaround time (TAT). Turnaround time definitions vary, but for the purposes of TGC, it should be from the time of specimen collection to the time the provider reviews the result ("vein to brain"). Based on the blood-glucose result, adjustment, if necessary, is then made to a continuous intravenous insulin infusion where dosing is adjusted on a set schedule (eg, every hour). To make this process work, blood-glucose testing performed at or near the bedside (or in the central laboratory with comparable turnaround time) is crucial. With many clinicians having turnaround time expectations of 30 to 60 minutes for central laboratory glucose results,[24] and with the laboratory limited by the time that it takes for a specimen to arrive, be registered, and be assayed, significantly shorter turnaround times (<30 minutes) for central laboratory testing may be possible but are unrealistic. Bedside results will always be generated, reported, and acted on in minutes as opposed to several tens of minutes. This makes central laboratory results impractical for TGC. However, point-of-care glucose testing (POCGT, bedside glucose) steps neatly into this role.

POCGT has always been beneficial to the diabetic inpatient by providing rapid blood-glucose results at mealtime so that insulin dosage can be modified as needed.[6,8] In addition, POCGT has also been a handy inpatient tool if an acute hypoglycemic episode is clinically suspected. Rapid turnaround time for POCGT has never been in an issue; however, there has never been solid evidence that POCGT actually improves patient outcomes. In fact, some have asked whether or not POCGT, with its increased cost relative to central laboratory,[25] is worthwhile. The evidence for POCGT is mixed. There is insufficient evidence for its use in routine care of the diabetic inpatient.[26] One could argue that POCGT was not absolutely necessary for quality patient care. However, there is potential evidence (based on the previously mentioned TGC studies) that a rapid blood-glucose result does improve outcome in the critical-care patient population. One could now argue that implementation of TGC protocols has finally provided an evidenced-based practice for the use of POCGT. It still remains to be determined whether or not POCGT methodologies can support TGC protocols. That is, are POCGT results sufficiently accurate and precise to support intensive insulin regimens?

Studies supporting the use of TGC have not been uniform in their methods section. Almost every manner of specimen type (whole blood, capillary, plasma, or serum), source (arterial, venule, or capillary [finger stick]), and collection method (finger stick, venipuncture, arterial line, and central venous catheter collection) has been used in studies of glycemic control. In addition, assay instrumentation has also varied from blood gas analyzers to one of several different types of handheld glucose meters. Often, specimen type and assay method have not been discussed or controlled for in the published studies of TGC (Scott MG, personal communication, 2009).[19] Discussion of the *Journal of the American Medical Association* 2008 TGC control study meta-analysis[17] showed that methods were only given in 10 of 27 studies[19] and, in those 10, there was no consistent assay methodology (Scott MG, personal communication, 2009).

That snapshot of protocols raises the possibility that blood-glucose measurement methods for TGC across all institutions vary just as widely. The same discussion raises the possibility that the inconsistency of the meta-analysis results was due to the variability in glycemic testing methods and problems associated with POCGT in the critical-care population. In the above-mentioned 2001 study, blood-glucose measurements were done on arterial blood samples on an arterial blood gas machine.[12] This indicates that concern was taken to standardize specimen type and assay method to eliminate that variable from the study.

Blood-glucose specimens for central laboratory testing are routinely venipuncture specimens (serum or plasma) that are centrifuged with testing performed on the noncellular ("plasma") component. In addition, several blood gas analyzer models are equipped to assay for glucose, if requested, on an uncentrifuged whole-blood specimen (arterial or venous). Testing for glucose by this method in the central laboratory is less common than the former method. POCGT encompasses a wide array of instruments ranging from handheld devices that assay single-use strips or cartridges to bench-top analyzers located near the patient (in unit-based satellite laboratories). Not surprisingly, there is a concomitant wide variety of methodologies in use.

POCGT is most often performed on a handheld device designed only for glucose analysis with a single-use media support intended for a small-volume whole-blood capillary specimen (collected by lancet of a finger tip [finger-stick specimen]). These devices have the longest history of use in point-of-care testing and have evolved to the point of being simple enough that any user can administer the test with a minimum of instruction. For this very reason, such tests have migrated out of the hospital and the licensed health care provider to diabetic patients for their own self-monitoring of blood glucose. Such tests have become important tools for diabetes management.[6–8] Because of the universality of such tests and because POCGT devices have become so easy to use, this article focuses on POCGT devices and their relation to TGC.

POCGT methodologies are currently based on one of several enzyme-coupled reactions (glucose oxidase, glucose dehydrogenase, or hexokinase) with a concurrent spectrophotometric or electrochemical measurement of reaction product to determine glucose concentration. The strip is a complex membrane that filters the whole-blood capillary specimen such that only the aqueous component (plasma or serum water) reaches the reaction site. At the reaction site, specimen glucose reacts with the enzyme used (dependent on vendor), producing a reaction product proportional to glucose concentration. In devices that use spectrophotometry, a colored product is generated in proportion to the glucose concentration. In those devices that use electrochemical methods, a current is generated proportional to the glucose concentration. The reader is referred to Nichols[27] for an excellent discussion of POCGT methodologies.

POCGT results are not interchangeable with those generated in the central laboratory. Laboratory (plasma) glucose results are 11% higher than whole blood glucose results because of differences in the aqueous components of cellular versus noncellular compartments of blood. Glucose freely diffuses in the aqueous component of blood and, because the plasma has a higher aqueous concentration, the concentration of glucose will be higher. Conversely, erythroctes contain less water per volume, so the concentration of glucose will be less. To address this issue, most POCGT devices have an 11% calibration factor such that results by device should match simultaneous ones assayed by the central laboratory.[27,28] This 11% calibration factor is set for a hematocrit of 45%. As a result, extremes of hematocrit can affect the POCGT result and should be evaluated during validation of new devices.

A number of other factors should be considered when interpreting POCGT results. For example, the user should know what is the general error of the devices and what causes it. POCGT has several unique sources of preanalytic and analytic error that will be discussed after a brief review of how much error is allowed.

Recommendations for POCGT analytic meter performance are listed in **Table 1**. Whether or not the recommendations are met can be elucidated from review of peer comparison data. College of American Pathologists 2008 glucose assay proficiency survey data[19] showed that central laboratory (29 methods, 5664 laboratories) coefficient of variations ranged from 2.5% to 4.3% compared with 12% to 14% for POCGT (17 methods, 19,957 sites). Bias results were also similar (no more than 11% difference between two central laboratory methods compared with no more than 41% difference between any two methods). In 2001, Boyd and Bruns[29] studied how bias and imprecision of POCGT devices affect insulin dosing. They pointed out that a total error of 5% would lead to an incorrect insulin dose 8% to 23% of the time and that a total error of 10% doubled the number of incorrect insulin doses (6%–45% of the time). They concluded that for the insulin dosing to be correct 95% of the time, bias and imprecision had to be less than 2%. Dhatt and colleagues[30] had better results in a 2004 study that evaluated glucose-meter performance for both experienced nurses and medical technologists. For the nurses, deviation from the American Diabetic Association criteria occurred 0% to 21% of the time. For medical technologists, deviations occurred 4% to 13% of the time.

Glucose concentrations can vary, depending on prandial state and collection site. Fasting glucose concentrations in capillary blood are slightly higher than in venous

---

Table 1
POCGT device analytical performance recommendations

Organization	Recommendation
American Diabetic Association	Initially proposed that total error should not be greater than 10% at glucose concentration between 1.7 and 2.22 mmol/L (30–400 mg/dL); total analytic error of <5% has been proposed, but no meter has yet achieved this
Clinical Laboratory Improvement Amendments of 1988 (CLIA)	Glucose meter results should be within 10% of target values or +/−0.3 mmol/L (6 mg/dL).
Clinical and Laboratory Standards Institute (CLSI) and the International Organization for Standardization (ISO) (2003)	For concentrations <4.2 mmol/L (75 mg/dL), <5% of samples should be +/−0.83 mmol/L (15 mg/dL) of the central laboratory result; for concentrations >4.2 mmol/L (75 mg/dL), <5% of samples should be +/−20% of the central laboratory result

Data from Sacks DB, Bruns DE, Goldstein DE, et al. Guidelines and recommendations for laboratory analysis in the diagnosis and management of diabetes mellitus. Clin Chem 2002;48(3): 436–72; Sacks DB, Arnold M, Bakris G, et al. Guidelines and recommendations for laboratory analysis in the diagnosis and management of diabetes mellitus: update (draft). Available at: http://www.aacc.org/members/NACB/LMPG. Accessed February 16, 2009.

blood, but the disparity between the two can show statistically significant differences (up to 70 mg/dL) in postprandial specimens. This is because the postprandial capillary specimens are glucose-rich while the venous specimens are glucose-poor postsystemic samples. Arterial and capillary specimens usually approach unity despite fed state.

As a function of the technology, two analytical problems specific to POCGT have been identified: (1) enzyme degradation and (2) effect of hematocrit.[6,31] Enzyme degradation secondary to improper storage of strips (eg, extremes of heat, cold, humidity) or use of expired strips with diminished effectiveness can affect results. The effect of patient hematocrit blood-glucose analysis has also been widely studied. Extremes of hematocrit can affect the POCGT result with elevated hematocrit associated with falsely lowered results and depressed hematocrit associated with falsely elevated results. Proposed mechanisms of interference include changes in specimen viscosity, mechanical impedance by erythrocytes at the level of the membrane filter, microclot formation, or protein deposition.[32,33] This hematocrit effect is independent of the plasma–whole-blood difference discussed earlier and, compared to the plasma–whole-blood difference, is not as well worked out without a calibration factor for correction.

Patient endogenous factors, such as pH or oxygen tension, can also affect results. For example, low oxygen tension, whether by hypoxia, shock, or decreased distal perfusion, impairs methods that use glucose oxidase.[6,31,34,35] Certain drugs have also been noted to affect POCGT results. Falsely elevated POCGT results have often been reported on patients on maltodextrin and ictodextrin. This interference has only been noted with instruments that use glucose dehydrogenase. Acetaminophen (glucose oxidase and glucose dehydrogenase), ascorbic acid (glucose oxidase and glucose dehydrogenase), dopamine (glucose dehydrogenase), and mannitol (glucose dehydrogenase) have also been noted to affect POCGT results.[31,36] The glucose strip itself is subject to analytic issues. Its most notable issue is its limitation for use only for the whole-blood capillary specimen.

The strip is designed for whole-blood capillary specimens. Use of other specimen types (arterial or venipuncture) has the potential to produce an erroneous result. Specific device instructions vary, but, in general, whole uncentrifuged blood is obtained via finger stick, followed by application of the blood drop to the strip, followed by insertion of the strip into the device. The logic of this approach is to make venipuncture unnecessary, therefore minimizing number of "sticks," as well as iatrogenic anemia. Unfortunately, in the intensive care patient with their plethora of catheters and frequent venipunctures for other laboratory testing, blood specimens are often acquired by many other means instead of finger stick. With strips designed for whole-blood capillary specimens, results from the use of specimens not vendor recommended become suspect. This issue becomes magnified in the critically ill patient population with their endemic variations in distal perfusion, hematocrit, and oxygenation status.

Multiple studies have looked at POCGT results in the critical-care population.[37–50] These studies looked at many variations of method comparison among different specimen types and assay methods. Point-of-care device versus central laboratory testing was the common theme for comparison (with some studies also looking at blood gas instrument glucose result as well). Finger stick (whole-blood capillary by point-of-care device) specimens were compared with simultaneous venous or arterial specimens (assayed on the point-of-care device, central laboratory instrument, or both).

The "cleanest" method comparison study of POCGT should consist of simultaneously collected arterial and finger-stick specimens. Use of a venous specimen is acceptable but is subject to the prandial difference discussed earlier. Arterial-specimen glucose results should be closer to results from specimens collected by finger stick. After collection, a temporally close (POCGT versus clinical laboratory analysis is then performed to minimize ex vivo glucose consumption. Of 12 identified studies that compared finger-stick to central laboratory testing, only 5 compared arterial specimens (assayed in the central laboratory and on POCGT device) to results generated using finger-stick specimens on the POCGT device.[39,41,42,45,46] For these 5 studies, most finger-stick glucose results did not correlate with central laboratory results. The tendency was for finger-stick results to be higher than those from arterial specimens; however, the converse was also identified is some studies. This finding was also seen with the remaining 7 studies. Although there are a limited number of studies, their discordance in conclusions lends weight to the hypothesis that POCGT may not be the appropriate methodology for TGC. One possible solution would be to decide which modality of testing is to be used (for a unit) and adhere to it. In this fashion, there would be an improvement in consistency of results by minimizing inter-specimen type and intermethod variability.

TGC involves use of an intensive insulin regimen based on frequent blood-glucose measurements to maintain blood glucose within a defined range. While evidence related to this practice has been inconsistent, the balance of evidence shows a definite improvement in morbidity and mortality. To make this process work in a practical sense, rapid glucose results are required, forcing a need for point-of-care (near bedside) glucose testing. However, there are limitations associated with point-of-care glucose that must be taken into account when using results generated in this fashion. Some key limitations are sensitivities to pH, oxygenation status, specific medications, and extremes of hematocrit. In addition to those factors, appropriate specimen type for analysis is also important to consider. Depending on instrument used, there can be significant differences between whole-blood via catheter (arterial/venous) specimens versus whole-blood via finger-stick (capillary) specimens, bearing in mind that the more common bedside glucose devices are designed for the latter class of specimen.

REFERENCES

1. Ravid M, Berkowicz M, Sohar E. Hyperglycemia during acute myocardial infarction. A six-year follow-up study. JAMA 1975;233(7):807–9.
2. Slingerland RJ, Fokkert M, Muller W, et al. Glycemic control and blood glucose monitors in hospitals. Point of Care 2005;4(4):150–3.
3. Stapleton RD, Heyland DK. Glycemic control and intensive insulin therapy in critical illness. In: Basow D, editor. Waltham (MA): Uptodate; 2009. Available at: http://www.uptodate.com. Accessed March 6, 2009.
4. McCowen KC, Malhotra A, Bistrian BR. Stress-induced hyperglycemia. Crit Care Clin 2001;17(1):107–24.
5. The effect of intensive treatment of diabetes on the development and progression of long-term complications in insulin-dependent diabetes mellitus. The Diabetes Control and Complications Trial Research Group. N Engl J Med 1993;329(14): 977–86.
6. Hirsch IB, Bode BW, Childs BP, et al. Self-monitoring of blood glucose (SMBG) in insulin- and non-insulin-using adults with diabetes: consensus recommendations for improving SMBG accuracy, utilization, and research. Diabetes Technol Ther 2008;10(6):419–39.

7. Montagnana M, Caputo M, Giavarina D, et al. Overview on self-monitoring of blood glucose. Clin Chim Acta 2009;402(1–2):7–13.

8. Standards of medical care in diabetes—2008. Diabetes Care 2008;31(Suppl 1): S12–54.

9. Langouche L, Van den Berghe G. Glucose metabolism and insulin therapy. Crit Care Clin 2006;22(1):119–29, vii.

10. Weintrob AC, Sexton DJ. Susceptibility to infections in persons with diabetes mellitus. In: Basow D, editor. Waltham (MA): Uptodate; 2009. Available at: http://www.uptodate.com. Accessed March 6, 2009.

11. Deedwania P, Kosiborod M, Barrett E, et al. Hyperglycemia and acute coronary syndrome: a scientific statement from the American Heart Association Diabetes Committee of the Council on Nutrition, Physical Activity, and Metabolism. Anesthesiology 2008;109(1):14–24.

12. Van den Berghe G, Wouters P, Weekers F, et al. Intensive insulin therapy in the critically ill patients. N Engl J Med 2001;345(19):1359–67.

13. Van den Berghe G, Wilmer A, Hermans G, et al. Intensive insulin therapy in the medical ICU. N Engl J Med 2006;354(5):449–61.

14. Ceriello A, Zarich SW, Testa R. Lowering glucose to prevent adverse cardiovascular outcomes in a critical care setting. J Am Coll Cardiol 2009;53(5 Suppl): S9–13.

15. Nesto R, Se I. Glycemic control for acute myocardial infarction in patients with and without diabetes mellitus. In: Basow D, editor. Uptodate. Waltham (MA): UpTo Date; 2009. Available at: http://www.uptodate.com. Accessed March 6, 2009.

16. Lazar HL, McDonnell M, Chipkin SR, et al. The Society of Thoracic Surgeons practice guideline series: blood glucose management during adult cardiac surgery. Ann Thorac Surg 2009;87(2):663–9.

17. Wiener RS, Wiener DC, Larson RJ. Benefits and risks of tight glucose control in critically ill adults: a meta-analysis. JAMA 2008;300(8):933–44.

18. Finfer S, Delaney A. Tight glycemic control in critically ill adults. JAMA 2008; 300(8):963–5.

19. Scott MG, Bruns DE, Boyd JC, et al. Tight glucose control in the intensive care unit: Are glucose meters up to the task? Clin Chem 2009;55(1):18–20.

20. Finfer S, Chittock DR, Su SY, et al. Intensive versus conventional glucose control in critically ill patients. N Engl J Med 2009;360(13):1283–97.

21. Inzucchi SE, Siegel MD. Glucose control in the ICU–how tight is too tight? N Engl J Med 2009;360(13):1346–9.

22. Moghissi ES, Korytkowski MT, Dinardo M, et al. American Association of Clinical Endocrinologists and American Diabetes Association Consensus statement on inpatient glycemic control. Endocr Pract 2009;15:1–17.

23. Hospital-acquired conditions. Available at: http://www.cms.hhs.gov/hospitalacqcond/. Accessed May 15, 2009.

24. Howanitz PJ, Cembrowski GS, Steindel SJ, et al. Physician goals and laboratory test turnaround times. A College of American Pathologists Q-Probes study of 2763 clinicians and 722 institutions. Arch Pathol Lab Med 1993; 117(1):22–8.

25. Howanitz PJ, Jones BA. Comparative analytical costs of central laboratory glucose and bedside glucose testing: a College of American Pathologists Q-Probes study. Arch Pathol Lab Med 2004;128(7):739–45.

26. Asrsand AK, Alter D, Frost SJ, et al. Diagnosis and management of diabetes mellitus. In: Nichols JH, editor. Evidence based practice for point of care testing. Washington, DC: AACC press; 2006. p. 44–62.

27. Nichols JH. Bedside testing, glucose monitoring and diabetes management. In: Kost GJ, editor. Principles and practices of point of care testing. 1st edition. Philadelphia: Lippincott Williams and Wilkins; 2002. p. 194–213.
28. D'Orazio P, Burnett RW, Fogh-Andersen N, et al. Approved IFCC recommendation on reporting results for blood glucose (abbreviated). Clin Chem 2005; 51(9):1573–6.
29. Boyd JC, Bruns DE. Quality specifications for glucose meters: assessment by simulation modeling of errors in insulin dose. Clin Chem 2001;47(2):209–14.
30. Singh Dhatt G, Agarwal M, Bishawi B. Evaluation of a glucose meter against analytical quality specifications for hospital use. Clin Chim Acta 2004;343(1–2): 217–21.
31. Dungan K, Chapman J, Braithwaite SS, et al. Glucose measurement: confounding issues in setting targets for inpatient management. Diabetes Care 2007;30(2): 403–9.
32. Tang Z, Lee JH, Louie RF, et al. Effects of different hematocrit levels on glucose measurements with handheld meters for point-of-care testing. Arch Pathol Lab Med 2000;124(8):1135–40.
33. Karon BS, Griesmann L, Scott R, et al. Evaluation of the impact of hematocrit and other interference on the accuracy of hospital-based glucose meters. Diabetes Technol Ther 2008;10(2):111–20.
34. Tang Z, Du X, Louie RF, et al. Effects of pH on glucose measurements with handheld glucose meters and a portable glucose analyzer for point-of-care testing. Arch Pathol Lab Med 2000;124(4):577–82.
35. Louie RF, Tang Z, Sutton Dv, et al. Point-of-care glucose testing: effects of critical care variables, influence of reference instruments, and a modular glucose meter design. Arch Pathol Lab Med 2000;124(2):257–66.
36. Tang Z, Du X, Louie RF, et al. Effects of drugs on glucose measurements with handheld glucose meters and a portable glucose analyzer. Am J Clin Pathol 2000;113(1):75–86.
37. Cook A, Laughlin D, Moore M, et al. Differences in glucose values obtained from point-of-care glucose meters and laboratory analysis in critically ill patients. Am J Crit Care 2009;18(1):65–71 [quiz 72].
38. Sylvain HF, Pokorny ME, English SM, et al. Accuracy of fingerstick glucose values in shock patients. Am J Crit Care 1995;4(1):44–8.
39. Slater-MacLean L, Cembrowski G, Chin D, et al. Accuracy of glycemic measurements in the critically ill. Diabetes Technol Ther 2008;10(3):169–77.
40. Ray JG, Hamielec C, Mastracci T. Pilot study of the accuracy of bedside glucometry in the intensive care unit. Crit Care Med 2001;29(11):2205–7.
41. Petersen JR, Graves DF, Tacker DH, et al. Comparison of POCT and central laboratory blood glucose results using arterial, capillary, and venous samples from MICU patients on a tight glycemic protocol. Clin Chim Acta 2008; 396(1–2):10–3.
42. Maser RE, Butler MA, DeCherney GS. Use of arterial blood with bedside glucose reflectance meters in an intensive care unit: Are they accurate? Crit Care Med 1994;22(4):595–9.
43. Marley JV, Davis S, Coleman K, et al. Point-of-care testing of capillary glucose in the exclusion and diagnosis of diabetes in remote Australia. Med J Aust 2007; 186(10):500–3.
44. Lacara T, Domagtoy C, Lickliter D, et al. Comparison of point-of-care and laboratory glucose analysis in critically ill patients. Am J Crit Care 2007;16(4):336–46 [quiz 347].

45. Karon BS, Gandhi GY, Nuttall GA, et al. Accuracy of Roche Accu-chek inform whole blood capillary, arterial, and venous glucose values in patients receiving intensive intravenous insulin therapy after cardiac surgery. Am J Clin Pathol 2007;127(6):919–26.
46. Kanji S, Buffie J, Hutton B, et al. Reliability of point-of-care testing for glucose measurement in critically ill adults. Crit Care Med 2005;33(12):2778–85.
47. Hoedemaekers CW, Klein Gunnewiek JM, Prinsen MA, et al. Accuracy of bedside glucose measurement from three glucometers in critically ill patients. Crit Care Med 2008;36(11):3062–6.
48. Finkielman JD, Oyen LJ, Afessa B. Agreement between bedside blood and plasma glucose measurement in the ICU setting. Chest 2005;127(5):1749–51.
49. Desachy A, Vuagnat AC, Ghazali AD, et al. Accuracy of bedside glucometry in critically ill patients: influence of clinical characteristics and perfusion index. Mayo Clin Proc 2008;83(4):400–5.
50. Critchell CD, Savarese V, Callahan A, et al. Accuracy of bedside capillary blood glucose measurements in critically ill patients. Intensive Care Med 2007;33(12):2079–84.

Fecal Occult Blood Testing

Kimberly W. Sanford, MD[a,*], Richard A. McPherson, MD[b]

KEYWORDS

- Colorectal cancer • Fecal occult blood testing
- Fecal immunochemical test • Fecal DNA test
- Colonoscopy • CT colonography

Colorectal cancer (CRC) is third most common cancer in the United States for both men and women. Approximately 150,000 newly diagnosed cases and 50,000 deaths attributed to CRC were projected for 2008. Overall, CRC accounts for 9% of all cancer deaths annually.[1] Fortunately, most of these deaths are preventable by a combination of screening and early treatment of precursor lesions. The survival rate for CRC is correlated to the stage at which the cancer is discovered. When the cancer is diagnosed at an early stage and remains localized, the 5-year survival rate is approximately 90%. When the cancer is diagnosed after regional metastasis to adjacent organs or lymph nodes, the survival rate decreases to 68%.[1] Early detection of CRC is essential to decreasing mortality.

The overall incidence of CRC has decreased over the last 20 years from 66.3 cases per 100,000 population in 1985 to 49.5 cases per 100,000 population in 2003. The sharpest decline in CRC occurred between 1998 and 2004, with a decreased incidence of 2.3% per year due to increased screening.[1] Mortality rates have also decreased over the past 2 decades, with the sharpest decline occurring between 2002 and 2004. During this time period, there was a 4.7% decrease in the mortality rate of CRC. This change reflects improvements in early detection and treatment of CRC.[1]

SCREENING FOR CRC

Most CRC arises in adenomatous polyps as a precursor lesion. The incidence of these polyps increases to as high as 30% in adults who are aged 50 years old and older.[2] Most patients remain asymptomatic until advanced disease is present. The symptoms of advanced disease are vague and include abdominal cramping and changes in

[a] Department of Pathology, Transfusion Medicine, Virginia Commonwealth University, 1200 East Marshall Street, P.O. Box 980231, Richmond, VA 23298, USA
[b] Division of Clinical Pathology, Department of Pathology, Virginia Commonwealth University, 1200 East Marshall Street, P.O. Box 980231, Richmond, VA 23298, USA
* Corresponding author.
E-mail address: ksanford@mcvh-vcu.edu (K.W. Sanford).

Clin Lab Med 29 (2009) 523–541
doi:10.1016/j.cll.2009.06.008
0272-2712/09/$ – see front matter © 2009 Elsevier Inc. All rights reserved.

bowel habits, and it is not until rectal bleeding begins that some patients seek medical attention. Due to the prevalence of disease and the presence of an identifiable precursor lesion, CRC is an ideal disease for screening in terms of cost effectiveness for early detection in addition to the overall benefit to individuals and to society as a whole.[3] Laboratory tests for screening large populations for a disease include the following characteristics: testing is inexpensive; the disease is detectable in an asymptomatic and preclinical stage; the disease can be prevented with medical intervention; the disease is prevalent in the population and creates a financial burden to society; and detection of disease has a benefit to the patient and society.[4]

Screening for CRC has demonstrated decreased mortality by identifying adenomatous polyps and localized malignant lesions that may be cured by surgical resection. One study demonstrated that if general population screening were performed, potentially 18,800 lives per year could be saved.[5] The Minnesota Colon Cancer Control Study was a randomized controlled study consisting of 46,551 participants ranging in age from 50 to 80 years.[6] The participants were randomly assigned to fecal occult blood testing (FOBT) annually, biennially (once every 2 years), or to a control group who had no screening performed. The study lasted for 13 years in which the screening group submitted six guaiac-impregnanted paper slides (Hemoccult) for each test event. Due to known interferences from dietary products, patients were instructed to stop ingesting red meat, poultry, fish, certain raw vegetables, fruits, aspirin, and vitamin C supplements for 24 hours before and during sample collection. The slides containing two smears from three consecutive bowel movements were mailed to the University of Minnesota Hospital where the testing was performed under a standardized and controlled procedure. Once received, 83% of the slides were rehydrated due to prolonged drying during transit in the mail system. If any of the six slides were positive for occult blood, the patient was urged to return to the hospital for follow-up studies which included a history and physical examination, routine laboratory tests, and colonoscopy.[6]

This study detected 1002 cases of CRC with 320 CRC-related deaths. Although the cumulative incidence of CRC was almost identical in the three groups, the cumulative annual mortality rate from CRC at 13 years was lower in the annually screened group (5.88/1000) than in the biennially screened group (8.33/1000), with the highest rate in the control group (8.83/1000). Overall, this study demonstrated a 33% decline in mortality in the annual screening group versus the control group (**Fig. 1**). Additionally, the study found a significant reduction in the incidence of higher grade cancer (Duke's stage D cancers). The study demonstrated a 48% reduction in these high grade cancers in a comparison with the control group.[6] The study also demonstrated a greater reduction in mortality than in three similar European studies demonstrating a decrease in mortality between 10% to 38% with FOBT screening.[7–13] The utility of screening is the detection of cancers that are readily removed before advancement to a stage D cancer. In this study, the 5-year survival rate was 2.4% in comparison with earlier stages, with 5-year survival rates of 94% for stage A, 84% for stage B, and 57% for stage C cancers.[6]

Interestingly, the biennially screened group only demonstrated a 6% decline in mortality rate when compared with the control group, which was not statistically significant. This finding appeared to be inconsistent with the benefit of annual screening and the 37% reduction in Duke's stage D cancers in the biennial group; therefore, the conductors of the study realized an extended follow-up may demonstrate a more significant reduction in mortality with biennial screening. A study performed in England demonstrated a 15% reduction in mortality and another study in Denmark demonstrated an 18% decrease in mortality with biennial screening.[14,15] Both of these studies demonstrated significant decreases in mortality with biennial screening. The

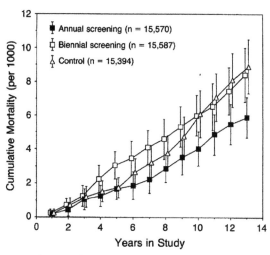

Fig. 1. Cumulative mortality in the annual screening group decreased by 33% when compared with the mortality in the biennial screening and control groups. (*From* Mandel JS, Bond JH, Church TR, et al. Reducing mortality from colorectal cancer by screening for fecal occult blood. N Engl J Med 1993; 328(19):1368; with permission.)

5-year, follow-up study to the Minnesota trial for a total period of 18 years demonstrated a 21% reduction in mortality for the biennially screened group. This observation was more consistent with other studies and also with the reduction of Duke's stage D cancers found in the earlier study.[16]

Multiple choices for noninvasive screening tests are now available for physicians and patients. Currently, recommendations by the American Academy of Family Physicians, the American Cancer Society, and the American College of Gastroenterology suggest that an average risk person should undergo CRC screening at 50 years old.[17-19] An average risk person is asymptomatic with no family or personal history of chronic inflammatory bowel disease, a strong family history of adenomatous polyps, or hereditary CRC syndromes. Anyone with an increased risk requires more intensive and frequent screening.[18,20] Currently, several screening test options are endorsed by the American Cancer Society (**Box 1**).

The FOBT and fecal immunochemical test (FIT) detect minute quantities of blood from precancerous and cancerous polyps which are detected by chemical or immunochemical methods. These tests should be performed annually; however, a single FOBT performed following digital rectal examination will miss approximately 95% of CRC and is not a recommended screening test.[21] The fecal DNA test is a new approach to CRC screening that uses molecular techniques to detect genetic mutations associated with the transition from adenomatous polyp to CRC. Currently, there is no recommended time interval to perform the stool DNA test.[20]

Some of the more invasive testing detects smaller polyps as well as cancer but is performed less frequently. Flexible sigmoidoscopy, double-contrast barium enema, and CT colonography (virtual colonoscopy) should be performed every 5 years. Colonoscopy is still considered the gold standard for screening because it allows for examination of the entire colon as well as the ability to biopsy or snare polyps during the procedure. The recommended interval for screening is 10 years. Because this invasive procedure carries the risk of perforation of the bowel or bleeding, the less invasive FOBT is more routinely performed.[21]

Box 1

American Cancer Society recommendations for CRC early detection in persons at average risk

Preventing CRC (and not just finding it early) should be a major reason for getting tested. Finding and removing polyps keeps some people from getting CRC. Tests that have the best chance of finding both polyps and cancer are preferred if they are available to you and you are willing to have them. Beginning at age 50 years, both men and women at average risk for developing CRC should use one of the following screening tests:

Tests that find polyps and cancer

Flexible sigmoidoscopy every 5 years: Colonoscopy should be done if test results are positive.

Colonoscopy every 10 years.

Double-contrast barium enema every 5 years: Colonoscopy should be done if test results are positive.

CT colonography (virtual colonoscopy) every 5 years: Colonoscopy should be done if test results are positive.

Tests that mainly find cancer

FOBT every year: Colonoscopy should be done if test results are positive. For FOBT or FIT used as a screening test, the take-home multiple sample method should be used. An FOBT or FIT done during a digital rectal examination in the physician's office is not adequate for screening.

FIT every year: Colonoscopy should be done if test results are positive. For FOBT or FIT used as a screening test, the take-home multiple sample method should be used. An FOBT or FIT done during a digital rectal examination in the physician's office is not adequate for screening.

Stool DNA (sDNA) test, interval uncertain. Colonoscopy should be done if test results are positive.

Reprinted with permission of the American Cancer Society.

SCREENING TESTS
FOBT by Guaiac Methods

The Dutch chemist Izaak van Deen was the first to recognize that when a natural resin from the *Guaiacum officinale* tree was mixed with blood and another reagent such as hydrogen peroxide, eucalyptus oil, or turpentine, the solution would turn blue. In 1958, Muller devised a way to impregnate paper with guaiac for detection of blood. In 1967, Greegor suggested coating paper slides with guaiac to perform FOBT at home.[6] Guaiac methods for the detection of occult blood (G-FOBT) are based on a chemical oxidation reaction between heme and alpha guaiaconic acid. The red blood cells released from the polyp or lesion contain hemoglobin as a major intracellular constituent. Hemoglobin consists of two pairs of polypeptide alpha and beta globin chains and four prosthetic heme groups, each containing one ferrous iron atom. The heme group has a pseudo-peroxidase activity that can catalyze the oxidation reaction of alpha guaiaconic acid, an active component in the guaiac paper, by hydrogen peroxide, the active component in the developer. This oxidation reaction will develop a highly conjugated blue quinone compound as illustrated in **Fig. 2**.[22]

Commercially available kits include single-slide test cards, double-slide test cards, or tape, all of which contain guaiac-impregnated paper. The Hemoccult single-slide test cards (Beckman Coulter, Fullerton, California) are most practical when only a single fecal sample is tested. Hemoccult II slides (Beckman Coulter) are provided to patients as a package of three tests. The patient collects stool specimens at home from bowel movements on three separate days. The patient returns the test

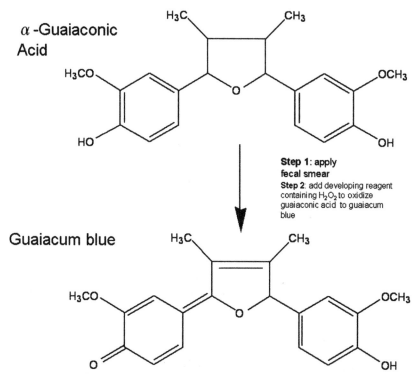

α-Guaiaconic Acid

Step 1: apply fecal smear

Step 2: add developing reagent containing H_2O_2 to oxidize guaiaconic acid to guaiacum blue

Guaiacum blue

Fig. 2. The chemical oxidation reaction of alpha guaiaconic acid for guaiac.

packs to the physician office for development and interpretation under controlled conditions. The Hemoccult Tape (Beckman Coulter) is suitable for in-office or bedside examination. Along with the guaiac-impregnated test cards or tape, there is also available developing solution, applicator sticks, instructions for the patient, and mailing pouches that are compliant with US Postal Service regulations as documented in the Federal Register for mailing clinical specimens.[23]

Patient preparation and instructions for G-FOBT are fairly extensive and require patients to abstain from particular foods and medications to prevent false-positive or negative results. Seven days before and during the stool collection period, patients should refrain from consuming non-steroidal anti-inflammatory drugs such as ibuprofen, indomethacin, and naproxen or more than 325 mg/d of aspirin. Use of these medications may induce slight bleeding in the stomach which can give rise to a positive test for blood in stool. Acetaminophen may be taken in place of these medications. Other medications capable of causing a false-positive test result include corticosteroids, phenylbutazone, reserpine, anticoagulants, antimetabolites, and chemotherapeutic drugs. Although they may turn stool black in color, iron supplements will not cause false-positive test results with G-FOBT.[23]

Other false-positive test results can occur from the consumption of particular foods. For 3 days before and during the stool collection, the patient should avoid all red meats including lamb, beef, and liver. Excessive alcohol intake can also cause false-positive tests results, presumably due to mild bleeding. Certain fruits and vegetables such as turnips and horseradish containing botanic peroxidases may also interfere with the oxidation reaction and lead to false-positive results;[24] however, evidence suggests that this dietary restriction is unnecessary because plant peroxidases naturally decompose within 72 hours, a time period that typically lapses before testing.[22]

One important cause of a false-negative result with G-FOBT is a high dose of vitamin C or ascorbic acid for at least 3 days before and during stool collection.[23,24] This artifact is due to the reducing properties of ascorbic acid, which interfere with the oxidation reaction between heme and alpha guaiaconic acid.[25] Patients should refrain from ingesting more than 250 mg/d of ascorbic acid. They should also refrain from ingesting excessive citrus fruits, juices, or other foods with excessive amounts of vitamin C. Also, any iron supplements containing more than 250 mg of ascorbic acid should be avoided.[23]

Any patient experiencing frank blood in the stool or gross hematuria should not collect a specimen for G-FOBT because it may represent another source of bleeding such as menstruation, urinary tract infection, or hemorrhoids. It is also recognized that povidone-iodine antiseptic preparations used to clean the perineal area must be washed thoroughly before stool collection. The iodine present in this antiseptic can cause a false-positive result with G-FOBT.[26]

Preparing and developing the G-FOBT

The patient collecting the sample should use the wooden applicator sticks provided with the kit to apply a thin smear of fecal sample to one of the two separate guaiac-impregnated slides. On the first slide, marked as A, the thin smear should cover the entire box. The same applicator is then used to sample stool from a separate area of the feces (using the other end of the applicator stick), and a thin smear is applied to cover the second slide labeled B. The cover flap is closed over the test slides which can be transported or mailed to the medical office or laboratory for processing.[23]

Delaying development of slides until 72 hours after sample application allows any naturally occurring peroxidases from vegetable material in the stool sample to decompose. The samples are stable for up to 14 days at room temperature (15–30°C) before developing. The test pack is flipped over, the back of the slide is opened, and two drops of developer containing 5% hydrogen peroxide are added to the guaiac paper directly over each smear. Results are read within 60 seconds; with the presence of any blue color, the test is interpreted as positive for occult blood. It is important that the developer have sufficient potency for test purposes. Accordingly, the bottle of developer should be capped between uses to prevent loss of hydrogen peroxide from decomposition. It is also significant for testing personnel to understand that the developer is not simply water despite its appearance and cannot be replaced with tap water. Drops of developer solution are also put onto positive and negative control areas of the slide to ensure integrity of the reactions and reagents. The positive area contains a hemoglobin-derived catalyst and will turn blue with the developer. Any blue color developed in the positive control area is interpreted as positive; however, the negative area should remain uncolored. The intensity or shade of blue color in the positive area should not be used as a positive reference for the patient sample. If the expected reactions with the performance monitor do not occur with the developer, patient test results are considered invalid.[23]

The Hemoccult II test is widely used and has a well-documented low sensitivity for detection of fecal occult blood and adenomas in asymptomatic patients with an average risk.[27,28] It was not until the Minnesota Colon Cancer Control Study was performed that the medical community realized FOBT could be used to decrease mortality caused by CRC. Rehydration of stool was performed because many of the samples spent prolonged times in transit to the testing center at the University of Minnesota. In this study, 82.5% of the slides were rehydrated by adding a drop of water to the guaiac slide before addition of the developer. As a result, a more than fourfold increase occurred in the rate of positive results and follow-up diagnostic tests.[6] Additionally, the readability of rehydrated tests can be unpredictable.[19] The rate of positive results increased from 2.4% to 9.8%, which was also correlated with the age of the patient. The rate of positivity with rehydration increased 8% in patients aged 50 to 59 years and 16% in patients aged 80 years and older. In comparison, the non-rehydrated slides did not demonstrate this same age trend. The positive rate for patients aged 50 to 59 years was 1.8% and the rate for patients aged greater than 80 years 2.4% with non-rehydrated slides. The positive rate was higher in men than women with slide rehydration. The sensitivity of the test increased from 80.8% to 92.2%; however, the specificity decreased from 97.7% to 90.4%. This loss of specificity also decreased the positive predictive value of the test from 5.6% to 2.2%.[6]

G-FOBT is designed to detect peroxidase activity of heme and hemoglobin. Red meat animal food products with a high heme content and plants with high peroxidase activity can cause a false-positive test result. Plant-derived peroxidase is believed to cause more false positives than heme from animal products. This difference may due to the fact that plant peroxidases have a higher enzymatic activity than hemoglobin owing to the differences in apoproteins and the observation that heme cannot survive the transit through the gut. Additionally, plant peroxidases are encased within an indigestible cellulose cell wall capable of surviving transit through the gut, causing false-positive results.[29]

The developer used in G-FOBT is an ethanol-based mixture with guaiaconic acid and hydrogen peroxide. The higher the ethanol concentration in the developer, the more likely the plant peroxidase will be denatured, causing less interference. Studies have demonstrated that higher water content of the fecal smear either by rehydration or by decreased drying time dilutes the ethanol concentration, resulting in a higher positive rate due to plant peroxidases.[6,28,29] Currently, rehydration of the slides is not a recommended procedure by Beckman Coulter, the US Preventive Services Task Force, and the American Gastroenterological Association.[19,23,30]

The two widely used FOBT tests are associated with a lack of certainty regarding which tests to use in different settings. The Hemoccult Sensa was compared with the Hemoccult II in five separate centers. Each center demonstrated a range of positivity; however, all studies concurred that the Hemoccult Sensa had a higher sensitivity rate than the Hemoccult (**Table 1**). This finding is most likely due to the fact that the Hemoccult Sensa has 5% more ethanol in the developer solution than the Hemoccult, which is more effective in denaturing the plant peroxidase activity.[29] Additionally, this change in the developer formulation allows for better stability and is more readable at the endpoint than in the Hemoccult. Multiple studies have demonstrated a better total positivity rate for the Hemoccult Sensa than the Hemoccult; however, the range of positivity is from 5% to 13.5%.[32–38] This wide range may be due to the length of time from specimen collection to development, the diets of subjects, or compliance with dietary restrictions. One study demonstrated a higher rate of positivity when patients ate red meat products within 3 days of performing G-FOBT, which became negative beyond 3 days.[39] Because the Hemoccult Sensa detects lower levels of hemoglobin, the sensitivity is increased. Additionally, another study demonstrated that if the fecal smear on the cards is left at room temperature for at least 48 hours before development, a diet high in plant peroxidases does not affect the results of the Hemoccult or Hemoccult Sensa test.[29]

Despite strong evidence that annual and semiannual G-FOBT screening improves mortality from CRC, there are three potential pitfalls. First, although the sensitivity of

Table 1
Comparison of CRC screening tests

Test Method	Advantages	Disadvantages	Sensitivity for Carcinoma (%)	Specificity for Carcinoma (%)	Cost ($)
G-FOBT	Inexpensive, widely available, studies demonstrate decreased mortality, no bowel preparation, noninvasive	Dietary and medication restrictions, low sensitivity and specificity, high number of false positives, must perform annually	12.9–54.2	95.2–97.5	3–4
FIT	Improved specificity, does not react with nonhuman hemoglobin, plant peroxidases, or upper gastrointestinal sources of bleeding, no bowel preparation, noninvasive	No epidemiologic studies demonstrating a decrease in mortality, no randomized controlled trials, may still have false-positive results, may miss lesions	87.5	96.6	18–30
Fecal DNA test	No bowel preparation, no dietary restrictions, noninvasive, collection performed at home	Expensive, not widely available, no epidemiologic studies demonstrating decrease in mortality, no recommended testing intervals, false-positive results	51.6	94.4	575
Colonoscopy	Visualize entire colon for lesions or inflammatory disease, diagnostic procedure for biopsy or removal of precancerous lesions for curative treatment	Bowel preparation required, invasive procedure with risk of perforation and hemorrhage, need to miss work, sedation, chaperone required	Gold standard for detection	Complete diagnosis by biopsy	1736
CT colonography[31]	Less invasive with lower risk of perforation over colonoscopy, identifies extracolonic abnormalities	Requires bowel preparation, radiation exposure, cannot detect lesions <1 cm	55–100	86–98	488

guaiac-based FOBT for detecting early cancer and adenomas greater than 1.0 cm in diameter is low, rehydration of the slides may increase sensitivity; however, this increase has led to an unacceptably high rate of false positives. Second, even though it is a screening test, the false-positive rate may be too high, leading to an unacceptably large number of diagnostic procedures. Third, G-FOBT is a more complicated procedure than other screening procedures due to the dietary restrictions and the collection requirement of multiple stool samples. To improve the screening process, multiple strategies have been suggested, including performing both the Hemoccult II and the Hemoccult Sensa or performing one of the G-FOBT tests in conjunction with an immunochemical for human hemoglobin in stool.[40]

Fecal Immunochemical Test

Due to the lack of specificity for hemoglobin in stool with G-FOBT, immunochemicals have been developed to serve as a screening test. These immunochemicals are capable of specifically detecting human hemoglobin, which eliminates the need for dietary restriction of red meat products and foods high in peroxidases. The FIT has increased sensitivity without excessive loss of specificity. There are no new trials reporting on mortality for this new screening method, although no studies have reported adverse effects of these higher sensitivity screening tests. Despite the lack of evidence supported by clinical trials, the use of any screening method is effective when compared with no screening.[41]

G-FOBT tests are designed to detect bleeding from upper and lower gastrointestinal sources. The FIT is more biologically selective in detecting colorectal bleeding and not bleeding from lesions proximal to the colon or distal small bowel.[42] The specificity of the test is based on the use of polyclonal antihuman hemoglobin antibodies that react with undegraded globin molecules in hemoglobin. Bleeding from sources proximal to the colon is exposed to bacteria and digestive enzymes which degrade the globin portion of hemoglobin such that the fecal sample would not react immunochemically with the FIT. Blood released from the distal small bowel or colon does not undergo this level of degradation; therefore, the globin molecule is capable of immunologically reacting with the FIT. This reactivity was well demonstrated in a study in which 10 healthy volunteers drank 20 mL of autologous blood on multiple days with subsequent collection of stool samples for both G-FOBT and FIT. All of the stool samples tested positive for occult blood with G-FOBT, but none tested positive by FIT.[43] Additionally, because FIT is specific for human blood in stool, there are no dietary or drug restrictions before stool collection, which improves participation with screening FOBT.[44] In fact, the only suggested patient preparation is increased consumption of roughage to increase the test sensitivity by detecting lesions that bleed intermittently.[45]

Test procedure

FIT has been approved by the US Food and Drug Administration for qualitative detection of fecal occult blood and has been endorsed by the American Cancer Society for CRC screening.[46] The principle behind one widely used FIT commercial kit involves sampling feces from two different areas of the stool. The stool is applied in a thin smear to a collection card, which is then transported to a testing site. The dried fecal smear is transferred to a test device card by using a pull-out sample tab. The sample is then rehydrated with a buffer solution containing sodium azide and bovine serum albumin. The test device is closed, bringing the sample in close contact with the test strip and initiating chromatographic flow of the sample. As the sample flows down the test strip, it rehydrates the colloidal gold antihuman hemoglobin conjugate. If human hemoglobin is present in the sample, an immune complex of human hemoglobin-conjugate is formed. This immune complex is captured on the test strip in a designated zone containing antihuman hemoglobin antibodies to form a visible test line, which is interpreted as a positive result. If the sample does not contain human hemoglobin, no test line forms, representing a negative result. Similar to the G-FOBT, there is a positive and negative control on each test device to ensure the reagents are appropriately reactive and the test was performed correctly. The unbound conjugate continues to migrate down the test strip to the positive control area which contains immobilized conjugate-specific antibodies. The positive reaction is indicated by a visible pink line color change; the test is considered invalid if there is no color change (**Fig. 3**). The negative control area located beneath the positive control will turn white or light pink, indicating conjugate has flowed through the test strip, but no test line forms. Patients are cautioned against using this test for 3 days before, during, or after their menstrual cycle. Also any patients with cuts on their hands, hemorrhoids, blood in their urine, or straining during defecation should not collect a stool sample. The test result should not be interpreted after 5 minutes

Step 1: Add rehydrated fecal specimen to test kit

Step 2: Sample flows down the test strip to rehydrate colloidal gold anti-human hemoglobin antibodies, forming immune complexes with free hemoglobin.

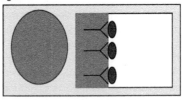

Step 3: Complex captured on test strip with anti-human hemoglobin antibodies to form a visible "test line" and unbound conjugate migrates to control line with contains conjugate specific antibody.

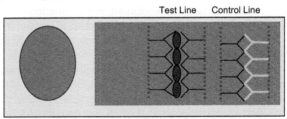

Fig. 3. Diagram of fecal immunochemical test. ——⟨, Anti-human hemoglobin antibody conjugate; ——⟨, Conjugate specific antibodies; ●, Human hemoglobin.

because this may result in a false-positive result.[45] Different manufacturers may use other conjugate materials such as latex.

Fecal immunochemical test compared with G-FOBT

Currently, there are no trials reporting on mortality for newer screening methods such as FIT;[41] however, studies comparing the performances of G-FOBT and FIT have demonstrated an increased sensitivity of FIT over G-FOBT. One of the most recent US studies enrolled 5841 patients with average risk for CRC. The study performed FOBT on the patients using high sensitivity G-FOBT (unrehydrated), FIT, and a combination of both tests over 2 years. The FIT detected 81.8% of invasive CRC compared with only 64.3% by the G-FOBT alone and the combination test. Similarly, the specificity for carcinoma by FIT was 96.9% compared with 90.1% for G-FOBT alone and 98.1% when both tests were used at the 95% confidence interval.[46] Another study demonstrated that FIT had a significantly better predictive negative and positive value than high sensitivity G-FOBT.[34]

A study from Germany compared six different FITs with one G-FOBT prospectively on 1319 participants of average risk for CRC. Performance characteristics were widely variable between tests. The overall positivity rate was lowest for the G-FOBT at 4.5% and ranged up to 46.4% for the Bionexia hemoglobin/hemopexin complex FIT. Test sensitivities for adenomas and advanced adenomas ranged from 11.4% to 58% and 25.4% to 71.5%, respectively. The sensitivities were slightly higher when patients with CRC and patients with advanced adenomas were combined. In particular, sensitivities for advanced adenomas ranged from 30% to 50% and specificities from 86% to 98%. The two best performing FITs (immoCARE-C [CARE diagnostica, Voerde, Germany] and FOB advanced [ulti med, Ahrensburg, Germany]) demonstrated sensitivities for advanced adenomas at 25% and 27% at the 95% confidence interval, respectively. The specificity for these assays was 97% and 93% at the 95% confidence interval, respectively. In comparison, the G-FOBT was 9.4% sensitive and 95.4% specific.[47,48] FIT could be a potential option for CRC screening in the future, considering it is easier to read and interpret the test results and has the same or better simplicity as G-FOBT for mass screening of populations. One editorial noted that any screening FOBT with a false-positive rate between 5% and 10% may still lead to excessive colonoscopy procedures.[40] FITs are two to five times more expensive than G-FOBTs, and this additional cost of screening may be too difficult to bear for some health care settings. Due to these increased costs, Medicare reimbursement rates are comparably five times higher for FIT ($23.22 per test) than for G-FOBT ($4.75 per test).[49]

Fecal DNA Testing

CRC develops sporadically, accounting for the majority of cases (approximately 85%), as a hereditary cancer syndrome, accounting for approximately 10%, or in the setting of inflammatory bowel disease. This progression from benign adenomatous precursor lesion to carcinoma is believed to occur over decades, allowing for accumulation of a series of sequential genetic alterations.[50] The progression to carcinoma occurs by either microsatellite instability (MSI) or chromosomal instability (CSI). Microsatellites are dinucleotide repeats, most commonly consisting of adenine and cytosine paired with thymidine and guanine, occurring thousands of times within the germline DNA. MSI is due to a gain or loss in the repeated units, resulting in a change in length. This alteration in length is only detected if many cells are affected by this same change, which is an indication of a clonal neoplasm. The loss of genes responsible for DNA mismatch repair results in the failure to detect when incorrect bases are inserted into a newly synthesized strand of DNA, leading to MSI. MSI is responsible for approximately 15% of CRC cases; these tumors are larger but associated with a more favorable prognosis. Other findings associated with MSI-induced CRC are that they are more commonly seen in younger patients with right-sided tumors which contain more mucinous features, are diploid, and have more lymphocytic infiltration. These carcinomas commonly have both synchronous and metachronous portions in the tumors.[51] The patients often have longer cancer survivals when compared with age-matched control patients with CSI, despite larger tumors with deeper penetration and poorly differentiated histology, although rarely are hepatic metastases identified.[52] Fecal DNA assays used to detect carcinomas stemming from MSI commonly use a marker to detect BAT-26, a repeat of 26 deoxyadenosines located in intron 5 of the MSH2 gene. BAT-26 is also a marker of long DNA, which is believed to represent disordered apoptosis of cancer cells as they are sloughed into the colonic lumen.[53] Variation in BAT-26 is a surrogate marker for CRC due to MSI.[54]

CSI causes approximately 85% of CRC, which is due to mutations occurring in both oncogene and tumor suppressor genes. These mutations accumulate in the adenomatous polyposis coli (APC) gene, p53 tumor suppressor gene, and the K-ras oncogene. CSI is characterized more by allelic losses as well as by chromosomal amplifications, translocations, and loss of heterozygosity. CSI is often referred to as the microsatellite stability pathway. Fecal DNA assays evaluating for the presence of CSI use markers detecting defects in the K-ras, APC, or p53 genes.[53]

The premise behind fecal DNA testing is that DNA markers are shed continuously by the exfoliation of epithelial cells lining the gut, in contrast to occult bleeding which is intermittent. As these cells are shed into the stool stream, the cells are degraded, releasing their DNA. Rapidly growing epithelial cells are continuously shed from adenomas and carcinomas which contain genetic mutations associated with colorectal neoplasias.[55] Because most adenomas do not bleed, this is an explanation for the low levels of sensitivities using G-FOBT to detect precursor lesions. One study demonstrated that many adenomas shed molecular markers that can be detected within the stool.[56]

Testing procedure

Patients are provided with plastic buckets which mount onto toilet seats. The patient is instructed to collect the entire bowel movement into the bucket without any urine, toilet paper, or other materials placed with the stool specimen. The sample bucket is removed from the toilet and placed in another container and into a provided cooler with a freezer pack to maintain a temperature of 0 to 4°C. The package is then mailed to the reference laboratory.[55]

Once the specimen is received in the reference laboratory, it is homogenized, and DNA is extracted from aliquots of homogenized stool after treatment with RNase. DNA fragments are purified by performing oligonucleotide-based hybrid capture assays for each CRC marker investigated. These purified DNA fragments are then amplified by real-time polymerase chain reactivity using target-specific primers targeting fragments 1.3, 1.8, and 2.4 from the capture sight. BAT-26 markers are analyzed by their size. Each polymerase chain reaction product is bound to a magnetic bead support, and a mutation-specific, solid-phase, mini-sequencing protocol identifies point mutations. All mini-sequencing products are analyzed by capillary electrophoresis with laser induced fluorescence detection. Each marker for mutation is assessed separately, and any patient with a positive marker for one of the mutations is considered positive for the fecal DNA tests. The patient is then instructed to consult with his or her clinician for appropriate follow-up testing.[53]

Fecal DNA test versus G-FOBT

Two recent studies have compared G-FOBT and fecal DNA testing. The earlier study evaluated 4400 asymptomatic patients aged more than 50 years with an average risk of CRC by fecal DNA testing. The fecal DNA testing detected 51.6% of cases with invasive carcinoma whereas G-FOBT identified only 12.9% of invasive carcinomas. In patients with invasive carcinoma or adenomas containing high grade dysplasia, the fecal DNA test detected 40.8% whereas G-FOBT identified 14.1%. In cases of adenomas, fecal DNA testing was able to detect 15.1% versus 10.7% by G-FOBT.[53]

A more recent survey of fecal DNA screening versus G-FOBT used two panels of gene targets for the fecal DNA tests. Test 1 contained 21 point mutations on the K-ras, APC, p53, microsatellite marker BAT-26, and long DNA. Test 2 contained point mutations on K-ras, the scanned mutator cluster region of APC, and vimentin methylation. Only the panel of mutations from test 1 was used in the Imperiale study.[53] In this study, the detection rates of neoplasms for test 1 were no better than with the G-FOBT, Hemoccult Sensa. In fact, the Hemoccult Sensa detected more cases of neoplasms than test 1. The stool DNA test 2 (SDT-2) did significantly better than the FOBT or the stool DNA test 1 (SDT-1). The SDT-2 detected adenomas at a rate three times higher than the SDT-1 for adenomas greater than or equal to 1 cm, four times higher than Hemoccult, and three times higher than Hemoccult Sensa. When compared with the markers present in SDT-1, the SDT-2 markers occur earlier in the adenoma to carcinoma progression, accounting for the higher rate of detection. It was concluded that all FOBTs are insensitive for the detection of adenomas owing to the fact that most adenomas do not bleed, but most shed neoplastic markers which can be detected in stool.[56]

Limitations of fecal DNA testing

A higher rate of positive test results occurs using the SDT-2 markers in patients with normal colonoscopies than with G-FOBT. This finding may be due to an increase in older patients.[56] There is a higher rate of K-ras mutations and methylated vimentin in the stool as we age without progression to CRC.[57] Also, DNA alterations may precede visible lesions, such as crypt foci with aberrant epithelium that are not detected by colonoscopy.[56] One editorial asks the question of whether fecal DNA should replace FOBT for mass screening of the population and supplies several reasons why it should not.[58] The first reason is the low sensitivity and specificity based on the study performed by Imperiale, demonstrating fecal DNA test sensitivity of 15% versus 11% when compared with G-FOBT and specificity of 94% versus 95% with G-FOBT.[53] The study by Imperiale only performed fecal DNA testing using SDT-1 markers; therefore, the outcome of the test results is directly impacted by the panel markers of genetic alterations selected.[53] The editorial by Woolf also raises the discussion of whether the health benefits of fecal DNA testing outweigh the harms. In the group aged 50 to 59 years, only 2% of patients with a positive fecal DNA test will have CRC upon colonoscopy; the remaining 98% of patients will have a negative colonoscopy and may continue to have anxiety that the colonoscopy failed to identify the lesion, and the DNA test could not be incorrect. Compliance may be low with this test because an entire bowel movement must be collected, stored, and shipped to the reference laboratory. Also, this test will most likely not be available to everyone because some health care plans will be unwilling to cover the expense.[58] Currently, this testing costs approximately $399, which is substantially higher than the cost of G-FOBT or FIT. Although there is now a CPT code available for this test, not all insurance carriers will approve performance of this test, and patients who want the test will have to self-pay. In response to the Imperiale study, one comment suggested that if fecal DNA testing were performed every 4 years, it would be less effective and less cost effective than performing colonoscopy examinations every 10 years.[59]

COMPLETE DIAGNOSTIC EVALUATION FOLLOWING POSITIVE FOBT

The previously mentioned trials demonstrated a significant decrease in mortality from CRC by performing annual or biennial FOBT by 33% and 21%, respectively.[6,16] Using FOBT as a primary screening tool for CRC, projected gains in life expectancy for US residents aged 50 to 54 years and 70 to 74 years, respectively, are 44 and 12 days using annual FOBT, 72 and 21 days using flexible sigmoidoscopy every 5 years, and 146 and 41 days using colonoscopy every 10 years.[3] These gains are of course calculated for the entire population; the individuals who actually have CRC detected and cured may have many years of increased survival. The success in these studies is based on greater than 80% of the patients with positive FOBT undergoing complete diagnostic evaluation.[60] Despite these convincing data, multiple studies demonstrate that only 34% to 59% of patients with positive FOBT undergo complete diagnostic evaluation.[61–65] Failure to undergo a complete diagnostic evaluation in these identified high risk patients is a serious lapse in health care because as many as 40% of patients with positive FOBT have large adenomas or CRC.[19,66] FOBT is only effective when colonoscopy is performed in patients who are positive.

There are myriad reasons why a complete diagnostic evaluation is not performed in patients who have a positive FOBT. Some of the reasons are a combination of the patient, the physician, and the systems in place. One study analyzed follow-up on 1041 patients with positive FOBT to determine whether a complete diagnostic evaluation was performed. The study found that 73% of the cases had a colonoscopy planned by the primary care physician, with colonoscopies completed in 62% of the cases. The largest single reason (7%) for not following up with colonoscopy was patient refusal. Other reasons why complete diagnostic evaluation was not performed included that the patient had left the practice (0.2%) and competing medical conditions (3%). The study also found that patients who were older than 80 years, younger than 50 years, uninsured, or had a colonoscopy within the previous 5 years were unlikely to follow-up with colonoscopy. Of all the colonoscopies performed, 29% revealed adenomatous polyps and 4% resulted in a diagnosis of CRC.[67] Another similar study demonstrated that 45% of patients with positive FOBT did not undergo complete diagnostic evaluation. In that study, 33% of patients did not undergo complete diagnostic evaluation because of a physician decision in which 19% of the reasons for nonperformance were compatible with published guidelines but 14% were not. Some of the documented reasons provided by physicians that were not compatible with published guidelines included the following: the patient had a flexible sigmoidoscopy performed, the patient's medical history suggested a possible reason for a positive test, the patient's age, lack of a positive family history, the finding that all three FOBT cards were not positive, or patient noncompliance with dietary or medication restrictions before FOBT.[60] A similar study surveyed 417 primary care physicians, of whom 85.1% offered CRC screening to their patients; however, only 51.8% would follow-up a positive FOBT with colonoscopy.[62] These studies suggest that physician education regarding the appropriate indications for complete diagnostic evaluation after a positive FOBT warrants more attention.

Currently, colonoscopy is regarded as the gold standard for screening because it has superior single test accuracy when compared with other CRC screening tests. Colonoscopy is also the final diagnostic test in the pathway to evaluate and treat patients with abnormal findings and allows for biopsy and polypectomy, which is curative in most cases. The procedure is invasive and presents a risk of complications, with an incidence of perforation of 3.8 in 10,000 cases, major bleeding in 12.3 of 10,000 cases, and other serious complications in 25 of 10,000 cases.[68] The procedure requires complete bowel preparation the day before the procedure, and patients undergo conscious sedation which requires missing a day from work and a chaperone for transport from the procedure. Colonoscopy is one of the most expensive screening assays, with median cost of $1736 in the United States.[68]

CT colonography, also referred to as "virtual colonoscopy," has excellent sensitivity of 55% to 100% and specificity of 86% to 98% in the detection of polyps greater than 1 cm; however, the accuracy for smaller polyps is much lower. The procedure also requires complete bowel preparation and air insufflation into the rectum through a rectal tube, but the risk of perforation is much lower than with traditional colonoscopy at 0 to 6 cases per 10,000 procedures. The rate of extracolonic findings is significant and ranges from 7% to 16% because it examines more than the interior of the colon.[68] The radiation exposure from this procedure is approximately 10 mSv per examination, and, currently, the potential risk of the low-dose radiation exposure is unknown. The impetus for the use of CT colonography is that it allows visualization of the colon with a lower risk of perforation and complication and may help reduce CRC mortality in patients who may otherwise refuse screening and would find this an acceptable alternative.

SUMMARY

A multitude of CRC screening tests are available with different levels of sensitivity and specificity; enrolling patients in one of these screening protocols improves their risk of mortality due to CRC. The testing ranges from a basic oxidation reaction catalyzed by hemoglobin resulting in a color change to detecting aberrant DNA from malignant epithelial cells as they are shed from the colonic mucosa. Advances in technology have led to increased costs for these screening tests without significant improvement in sensitivity or specificity for CRC. Currently, colonoscopy is used as the gold standard for screening tests as well as the complete diagnostic test plus definitive treatment for many patients. Compliance with colonoscopy is suboptimal because of the patient preparation and risk associated with the invasive procedure. Virtual colonoscopy is a newly introduced screening and diagnostic test that has a lower risk and is less invasive than a traditional colonoscopy; however, it is less sensitive for precursor lesions less than 1 cm. Future studies will determine the acceptability of these newer screening tests and result in an eventual decrease in pricing of this advanced technology.

REFERENCES

1. Cancer facts & figures 2008. Atlanta (GA): American Cancer Society; 2008. Available at: http://www.cancer.org/downloads/STT/2008CAFFfinalsecured.pdf. Accessed March 28, 2009.
2. Rickert RR, Auerbach O, Garfinkel L, et al. Adenomatous lesions of the large bowel: an autopsy survey. Cancer 1979;43(5):1847–57.
3. Inadomi JM. Taishotoyama Symposium Barriers to colorectal cancer screening: economics, capacity and adherence. J Gastroenterol Hepatol 2008;23(Suppl 2):S198–204.
4. Glenn GC. Practice parameter on laboratory panel testing for screening and case finding in asymptomatic adults. Arch Pathol Lab Med 1996;120:929–43.

5. Maciosek MV, Solberg LI, Coffield AB, et al. Colorectal cancer screening: health impact and cost effectiveness. Am J Prev Med 2006;31(1):80–9 [PMID: 16777546].

6. Mandel JS, Bond JH, Church TR, et al. Reducing mortality from colorectal cancer by screening for fecal occult blood. N Engl J Med 1993;328(19):1365–71.

7. Kewenter J, Bjork S, Haglind E, et al. Screening and rescreening for colorectal cancer: a controlled trial of fecal occult blood testing in 27,700 subjects. Cancer 1988;62:645–51.

8. Klaaborg K, Madsen MS, Sondergaard O, et al. Participation in mass screening for colorectal cancer with fecal occult blood test. Scand J Gastroenterol 1986; 21:1180–4.

9. Kronborg O, Fenger C, Sondergaard O, et al. Initial mass screening for colorectal cancer with fecal occult blood test: a prospective randomized study at Funen in Denmark. Scand J Gastroenterol 1987;22:677–86.

10. Kronborg O, Fenger C, Olsen J, et al. Repeated screening for colorectal cancer with fecal occult blood test: a prospective randomized study at Fenen, Denmark. Scand J Gastroenterol 1989;24:599–606.

11. Kronborg O, Fenger C, Worm J, et al. Causes of death during the first 5 years of a randomized trial of mass screening for colorectal cancer with fecal occult blood test. Scand J Gastroenterol 1992;27:47–52.

12. Hardcastle JD, Farrands PA, Balfour TW, et al. Controlled trial of faecal occult blood testing in the detection of colorectal cancer. Lancet 1983;2:1–4.

13. Hardcastle JD, Farrands PA, Balfour TW, et al. Randomised, controlled trial of faecal occult blood screening for colorectal cancer: results for first 107,349 subjects. Lancet 1989;1:1160–4.

14. Kronborg O, Fenger C, Olsen J, et al. Randomised study of screening for colorectal cancer with faecal occult blood test. Lancet 1996;348:1472–7.

15. Hardcastle JD, Chamberlain JO, Robinson MHE, et al. Randomised controlled trial of faecal occult blood screening for colorectal cancer. Lancet 1996;348: 1472–7.

16. Mandel JS, Church TR, Ederer R, et al. Colorectal cancer mortality: effectiveness of biennial screening for fecal occult blood. J Natl Cancer Inst 1999;91(5):434–7.

17. American Academy of Family Physicians. A-E recommendations for clinical preventive services. Available at:http://www.aafp.org/online/en/home/clinical/exam/a-e.html. Accessed March 28, 2009.

18. American Cancer Society guidelines for the early detection of cancer. Available at: http://www.cancer.org/docroot/ped/content/ped_2_3x_acs_cancer_detection_guidelines_36.asp. Accessed March 28, 2009.

19. Winawer S, Fletcher R, Rex D, et al. Colorectal cancer screening and surveillance: clinical guidelines and rationale–update based on new evidence. Gastroenterology 2003;124:544–60.

20. Wilkins T, Reynolds PL. Colorectal cancer: a summary of the evidence for screening and prevention. Am Fam Physician 2008;78(12):1385–92.

21. Pignone M, Rich M, Teutsch SM, et al. Screening for colorectal cancer in adults at average risk: a summary of the evidence for US Preventative Services Task Force. Ann Intern Med 2002;137(2):132–41.

22. Kratochvil JF, Burriss RH, Seikel MK, et al. Isolation and characterization of alpha-guaiaconic acid and the nature of guaiacum blue. Phytochemistry 1971;10:2529.

23. Beckman Coulter. Hemoccult product instruction Available at:http://www.beckmancoulter.com/literature/ClinDiag/462478-E_HO.pdf. Updated September 2003. Accessed March 28, 2009.

24. Ouyang D, Chen J, Getzenberg R, et al. Noninvasive testing for colorectal cancer: a review. Am J Gastroenterol 2005;100:1393–403.
25. Jaffe RM, Kasten B, Young DS, et al. False-negative stool occult blood tests caused by ingestion of ascorbic acid (vitamin C). Ann Intern Med 1975;83: 824–6.
26. Blebea J, McPherson RA. False-positive guaiac testing with iodine. Arch Pathol Lab Med 1985;109:437–40.
27. Allison JE, Feldman R, Tekawa IS. Hemoccult screening in detecting colorectal neoplasm: sensitivity, specificity, and predictive value. Long-term follow-up in a large group practice setting. Ann Intern Med 1990;112(5):328–33.
28. Ahlquist DA, Wieand HS, Moertel CG, et al. Accuracy of fecal occult blood screening for colorectal neoplasia: a prospective study using Hemoccult and HemoQuant tests. JAMA 1993;269:1262–7.
29. Sinatra MA, St. John JB, Young GP. Interference of plant peroxidases with guaiac-based fecal occult blood tests is avoidable. Clin Chem 1999;45(1):123–6.
30. US Preventative Services Task Force. Screening for colorectal cancer recommendation and rationale. Ann Intern Med 2002;137(2):96–104.
31. Zauber AG, Knudsen AB, Rutter CM, et al. Cost-effectiveness of CT colonography to screen for colorectal cancer. Rockville (MD): Agency for Healthcare Research and Quality; 2009. Technology Assessment Report Project ID: CTCC0608. Available at: http://www.cms.hhs.gov/determinationprocess/downloads/id58TA.pdf. Accessed March 31, 2009.
32. Levin B, Hess K, Johnson C. Screening for colorectal cancer: a comparison of 3 fecal occult blood tests. Arch Intern Med 1997;157:970–6.
33. Rozen P, Knaani J, Samuel Z. Comparative screening with a sensitive guaiac and specific immunochemical occult blood test within an endoscopy study. Cancer 2000;89(1):46–52.
34. St John DJB, Young GP, Alexeyett MA, et al. Evaluation of new occult blood tests for detection of colorectal neoplasia. Gastroenterology 1993;104:1661–8.
35. Petrelli N, Michalek AM, Freedman A, et al. Immunochemical versus guaiac occult blood stool tests: results of a community based screening program. Surg Oncol 1994;3:27–36.
36. Rozen P, Knaani J, Papo N. Evaluation and comparison of an immunochemical and a guaiac faecal occult blood-screening test for colorectal neoplasia. Eur J Cancer Prev 1995;4:475–81.
37. Rozen P, Knaani J, Samuel Z. Performance characteristics and comparison of two immunochemical and two guaiac fecal occult blood screening tests for colorectal neoplasia. Dig Dis Sci 1997;42(10):2064–71.
38. Allison JE, Tekawa IS, Ransom LJ. A comparison of fecal occult blood tests for colorectal cancer screening. N Engl J Med 1996;334(3):155–9.
39. Feinberg EJ, Steinberg WM, Banks B, et al. How long to abstain from eating red meat before fecal occult blood tests. Ann Intern Med 1990;113:403–4.
40. Ransohoff DF, Lang CA. Improving the fecal occult blood test. N Engl J Med 1996;334(3):189–90.
41. US Preventative Services Task Force. Screening for colorectal cancer recommendation statement. Ann Intern Med 2008;149(9):627–37.
42. Young GP, John JB, Winawer SJ, et al. Choice of fecal occult blood tests for colorectal cancer screening: recommendations based on performance characteristics in population studies. Am J Gastroenterol 2002;97(10):2499–506.
43. Rockey DC, Auslander A, Greenberg PD. Detection of upper gastrointestinal blood with fecal occult blood tests. Am J Gastroenterol 1999;94:344–50.

44. Cole SR, Young GP. Effect of dietary restriction on participation in faecal occult blood test-based screening for colorectal cancer. Med J Aust 2001;175(4): 195–8.

45. Beckman Coulter. Hemoccult ICT immunochemical fecal occult blood test product instructions. Updated June 2005. Available at:http://www.beckmancoulter.com/literature/ClinDiag/1_395069-F.pdf. Accessed March 28, 2009.

46. Imperiale T. Quantitative immunochemical fecal occult blood tests: is it time to go back to the future [editorial]? Ann Intern Med 2007;146(4):309–11.

47. Allison JE, Sakoda LC, Levin TR, et al. Screening for colorectal neoplasms with new fecal occult blood tests: update on performance characteristics. J Natl Cancer Inst 2007;99:1462–70.

48. Hundt S, Haug U, Brenner H. Comparative evaluation of immunochemical fecal occult blood tests for colorectal adenoma detection. Ann Intern Med 2009; 150(3):162–9.

49. CodeMap national for 2008 laboratory fees. Available at:https://www.codemap.com/ivd/userhome.cfm. Accessed March 28, 2009.

50. Fearon E, Vogelstein B. A genetic model for colorectal tumorigenesis. Cell 1990; 61:759–67.

51. Soreide K, Janssen EA, Soiland H, et al. Microsatellite instability in colorectal cancer. Br J Surg 2006;93:395–406.

52. Gryfe R, Kim H, Hsieh ETK, et al. Tumor microsatellite instability and clinical outcome in young patients with colorectal cancer. N Engl J Med 2000;342: 69–77.

53. Imperiale T, Ransohoff DF, Itzkowitz SH, et al. Fecal DNA versus fecal occult blood for colorectal cancer screening in an average-risk population. N Engl J Med 2004;351(26):2704–14.

54. Hoang JM, Cottu PH, Thuille B, et al. BAT-26, an indicator of the replication error phenotype in colorectal cancers and cell lines. Cancer Res 1997;57:300–3.

55. DNA Direct. DNA stool testing with DNA Direct. Available at:http://www.dnadirect.com. Accessed March 28, 2009.

56. Ahlquist DA, Sargent DJ, Loprinzi CL, et al. Stool DNA and occult blood testing for screen detection of colorectal neoplasia. Ann Intern Med 2008; 149(7):441–50.

57. Chien CC, Chen SH, Liu CC, et al. Correlation of K-ras codon 12 mutations in human feces and ages of patients with colorectal cancer (CRC). Transl Res 2007;149:96–102.

58. Woolf S. A smarter strategy? Reflections on fecal DNA screening for colorectal cancer. N Engl J Med 2004;351(26):2755–8.

59. Frossard JL, Peyer R. Fecal DNA for colorectal cancer screening. N Engl J Med 2005;352(13):1384–5.

60. Jimbo M, Myers RE, Hyslop T, et al. Reasons patients with a positive fecal occult blood test result do not undergo complete diagnostic evaluation. Ann Fam Med 2009;7(1):11–6.

61. Myers RE, Balshem AM, Wolf TA, et al. Screening for colorectal neoplasia: physicians' adherence to complete diagnostic evaluation. Am J Public Health 1993; 83(11):1620–2.

62. Sharma VK, Vasudeva R, Howden CW. Colorectal cancer screening and surveillance practices by primary care physicians: results of a national survey. Am J Gastroenterol 2000;95(6):1551–6.

63. Lurie JD, Welch HG. Diagnostic testing following fecal occult blood screening in the elderly. J Natl Cancer Inst 1999;91:1641–6.

64. Shields HM, Weiner MS, Henry DR, et al. Factors that influence the decision to do an adequate evaluation of a patient with a positive stool for occult blood. Am J Gastroenterol 2001;96(1):196–203.
65. Ko CW, Dominitz JA, Nguyen TD. Fecal occult blood testing in a general medical clinic: comparison between guaiac-based and immunochemical based tests. Am J Med 2003;115(2):111–4.
66. Ransohoff DF, Lang CA. Screening for colorectal cancer with the fecal occult blood test: a background paper. American College of Physicians. Ann Intern Med 1997;126:811–22.
67. Rao SK, Schilling TF, Sequist TD. Challenges in the management of positive fecal occult blood tests. J Gen Intern Med 2009;24(3):356–60.
68. Whitlock EP, Lin JS, Lilies E, et al. Screening for colorectal cancer: an updated systematic review. Evidence synthese no. 65, part 1. AHRQ publication no. 08-05124-EF-1. Rockville (MD): Agency for Healthcare Research and Quality; 2008.

Point-of-Care Testing
in Coagulation

Elizabeth M. Van Cott, MD

KEYWORDS

- D-dimer • PT/INR • Platelet function testing
- Activated clotting time

Point-of-care (POC) assays are available for a variety of coagulation tests. These assays are generally simple to perform and have a more rapid turnaround time than their central-laboratory counterparts. In this article, the current status of coagulation POC methodologies is discussed, focusing the potential clinical uses and the limitations of platelet function testing, prothrombin time/international normalized ratio (INR), D-dimer, and activated clotting time (ACT). Platelet function POC tests are receiving growing attention, but their clinical role is yet to be defined. Prothrombin time/INR POC testing has limitations but, under certain conditions, is proposed to be suitable for patient self-testing in the management of outpatient anticoagulation therapy. D-dimer POC tests are available, but their suitability for the exclusion of venous thromboembolism (VTE) remains to be established. ACT testing remains a commonly used bedside test for rapid monitoring of high-doses of heparin anticoagulation. Activated partial thromboplastin time (PTT) POC tests are also commercially available but are not discussed herein, because the demand for PTT POC testing has been low and the reliability of their results has remained in question.[1]

PLATELET FUNCTION POINT-OF-CARE TESTING

Platelet aggregation with a platelet aggregometer is the gold standard for platelet function testing, but this method is labor-intensive and requires laboratory technologist expertise; therefore, it is not well suited for high-volume, rapid testing. In recent years, rapid devices that can be used in the laboratory or at the POC have become available, but the results do not always correlate well with platelet aggregation[2] (and with unpublished observations), and more studies are needed to determine the role of these new devices.[3]

One device that is commonly in use is the platelet function analyzer PFA-100 (Siemens Corporation, New York, New York). According to the College of American Pathologists proficiency survey PF-A 2009, more than 900 laboratories are using this device. A number of laboratories are using another POC device called

Department of Pathology, Massachusetts General Hospital, Gray-Jackson 235, 55 Fruit Street, Boston, MA 02114, USA

Clin Lab Med 29 (2009) 543–553
doi:10.1016/j.cll.2009.06.016
0272-2712/09/$ – see front matter © 2009 Elsevier Inc. All rights reserved.

Plateletworks (Helena Laboratories, Beaumont, Texas). The PFA-100 measures the time in seconds that it takes to occlude a channel that is coated with collagen and ADP or collagen and epinephrine (which activate platelets) as the patient's whole-blood sample flows through the channel. Required for each test is 800 μL citrated whole blood (ie, 1600 μL to perform the ADP and the epinephrine cartridge). The International Society on Thrombosis and Haemostasis (ISTH) noted that PFA-100 results are often abnormal in a variety of congenital platelet function disorders, but the device is not sensitive enough to be used as a screening test to exclude such disorders.[3] Studies have shown that PFA-100 results are abnormal in many cases of moderate or severe von Willebrand's disease, but the test is not as sensitive for detecting mild cases.[4] A prospective study reported that short baseline ADP closure time (72 seconds) at the time of ST-elevation myocardial infarction (MI), before therapy, was associated with an increased risk of major adverse cardiac outcomes during 2-year follow-up. Baseline epinephrine closure time was not associated with clinical outcome.[5]

Some POC devices are intended for (or have been investigated for) monitoring anti-platelet medications such as aspirin, clopidogrel, or glycoprotein IIb/IIIa inhibitors, but results from the various methods generally do not have strong agreement with platelet aggregation or with each other. In one study, compared with platelet aggregation, the PFA-100 was 62% sensitive and VerifyNow (Accumetrics, San Diego, California) was 39% sensitive in detecting "aspirin resistance."[2] The ISTH recommended against performing platelet function tests to assess, monitor, or adjust dosing of aspirin therapy.[3,6] Consensus guidelines from the American College of Chest Physicians (ACCP) note that the clinical relevance of laboratory testing for aspirin resistance remains to be established, and "no test of platelet function is recommended to assess the antiplatelet effect of aspirin" at this time.[7] These guidelines also do not recommend performing platelet function tests to assess the effects of aspirin, clopidogrel, or other antiplatelet agents before surgery, because the methods are not well studied for most types of surgery, the significance of the results is uncertain, and the results have not identified patients at increased risk for surgical bleeding.[8] Aspirin doses above 75 to 81 mg daily do not seem to improve prevention of cardiovascular disease but do increase the risk for bleeding.[9]

Using gold standard platelet aggregation, a typical definition of aspirin resistance is greater than 20% aggregation with arachidonate,[10] but other definitions use collagen or ADP aggregation. One definition of clopidogrel resistance is 50% aggregation or higher with 5 μM ADP[11] or 70% or higher with 10 μM ADP,[12] but this is not well-defined and other definitions have also been used. These prospective studies found an association between aspirin[10] or clopidogrel[11,12] resistance and increased adverse cardiovascular outcomes.

Some prospective studies have also been reported for some of the POC devices—in particular, the PFA-100 and Accumetrics devices. Accumetrics offers POC testing for aspirin, clopidogrel, or glycoprotein IIb/IIIa platelet inhibition. In patients who have stable coronary artery disease, aspirin-resistant patients (as defined by the Accumetrics device) had a significantly higher rate of adverse cardiovascular outcomes after 1 year of follow-up than patients who did not have aspirin resistance.[13] In contrast, Buch and colleagues[14] found no relation between the Accumetrics result for aspirin and creatine kinase–MB or troponin I after percutaneous coronary intervention (PCI), nor with clinical outcome at 6 months. Studying clopidogrel with the Accumetrics device, Price and colleagues[15] found that patients undergoing drug-eluting stent implantation with a platelet reactivity of 235 P2Y12 reaction units (PRUs) or greater on clopidogrel had significantly more stent thrombosis and cardiovascular death within

6 months after the procedure. This cutoff was 78% sensitive and 68% specific, with 99% negative predictive value (NPV) in predicting 6-month outcomes. Marcucci and colleagues[16] reported that 240 PRUs or greater on clopidogrel was significantly associated with cardiovascular death and nonfatal MI, but there was no association with target-vessel revascularization. The 240 PRU cutoff was 61% sensitive and 70% specific, with 96% NPV in predicting cardiovascular death or nonfatal MI at 12 months.[16] In addition, with the Accumetrics device, patients who had the highest quartile of clopidogrel platelet reactivity before PCI were associated with an increased risk of cardiac death, MI, or target-vessel revascularization at 30 days post PCI.[17] In contrast, clopidogrel platelet reactivity at 8 or 24 hours after PCI had no association with these cardiac outcomes.[17] Buch and colleagues[14] found no relation between the Accumetrics result for clopidogrel and creatine kinase–MB or troponin I after PCI, nor with clinical outcome at 6 months.

The PFA-100 does not appear to be significantly affected by clopidogrel[3] and is therefore generally not used to assess clopidogrel effect. A new cartridge designed to detect clopidogrel effect on the PFA-100 is in development. In contrast, aspirin typically prolongs the epinephrine closure time on the PFA-100 (with normal ADP closure time); therefore, some prospective studies were conducted using the PFA-100 to assess for aspirin resistance. Gianetti and colleagues[18] reported that epinephrine closure times of less than 190 seconds or the lowest quartile of ADP closure times had a significantly increased rate of recurrence of coronary events within 6 months after PCI. Marcucci and colleagues[19] reported similar findings using a cutoff of less than 203 seconds with the epinephrine cartridge. Two other studies did not find a significant difference in outcomes between aspirin-resistant and -sensitive coronary artery disease patients, using a cutoff of less than 196 seconds and less than 186 seconds, respectively (although a nonsignificant trend was noted).[20,21]

Causes of aspirin or clopidogrel resistance are not completely understood but appear to be multifactorial. Clopidogrel is an inactive prodrug that must be metabolized into an active form by cytochrome P-450 (CYP) enzymes in the liver. Certain CYP polymorphisms (in the gene CYP2C19) or polymorphisms of ABCB1 (a gene that is necessary for clopidogrel absorption) have recently been associated with adverse cardiac outcomes.[22,23] Omeprazole has often been admininstered to patients receiving clopidogrel and aspirin to protect against gastrointestinal bleeding complications, but there is recent evidence that the use of omeprazole with clopidogrel is associated with an increased risk of death or rehospitalization for acute coronary syndrome compared to clopidogrel alone,[24] possibly because omeprazole might inhibit the activation of clopidogrel by inhibiting CYP2C19.[25] When a nonsteroidal anti-inflammatory drug (NSAID) such as ibuprofen is taken before aspirin, the NSAID can cause aspirin resistance. The NSAID binds temporarily to cyclooxygenase-1 (COX-1), preventing aspirin from binding. Although aspirin, when it binds to COX-1, irreversibly inactivates the platelet, the active form of aspirin has a half-life of only approximately 15 to 20 minutes. Therefore, by the time the NSAID is cleared and COX-1 is available for binding, the aspirin is no longer present. Acute-phase reactions with elevations of acute-phase-reactant proteins, particularly von Willebrand's factor, can shorten PFA-100 closure times,[3] giving the appearance of aspirin resistance. Various other causes of aspirin resistance are known or are proposed to exist.

PFA-100 closure times are prolonged by low platelet counts, low hematocrit, glycoprotein IIb/IIIa inhibitors, and paroxetine (a serotonin-reuptake inhibitor).[3] Red wine or chocolate can prolong the epinephrine closure time.[3] Hemolyzed specimens are not recommended.

Accumetrics results for aspirin and clopidogrel are influenced by low hematocrit, low platelet count, and glycoprotein IIb/IIIa inhibitors. In addition, the aspirin assay is also influenced by NSAIDs.

To determine the clinical utility, if any, of these tests, prospective randomized trials assessing for an association between platelet function test results and clinical outcomes are needed. In addition, it is not known whether altering therapy on the basis of platelet function tests is of any benefit. It also is too soon to know whether there is a role for genetic testing for polymorphisms that affect clopidogrel metabolism.[26]

PROTHROMBIN TIME/INTERNATIONAL NORMALIZED RATIO POINT-OF-CARE TESTING

Several POC INR devices are available for monitoring oral anticoagulant therapy, of which some are intended for professional use and others are designed for patient self-testing. Patient self-testing expenses are at least partly reimbursable through Medicare. The amount of blood required to perform a POC INR is very small (typically $\leq 50\ \mu L$) compared with testing in a traditional laboratory (typically $\geq 1.8\ mL$). Although the quality of current POC devices is improved over older models,[1] discrepancies between POC devices and laboratory INRs still exist.[27,28]

CoaguChek S (Roche Diagnostics, Indianapolis, Indiana),[28–30] for professional use, is being replaced by CoaguChek XS, for professional use or patient self-testing.[28,29,31,32] Devices for patient self-testing that are approved by the Food and Drug Administration are CoaguChek XS, INRatio2 (Hemosense Inc, San Jose, California), and ProTime 3 or the newer model, New ProTime (International Technidyne Corporation, Edison, New Jersey). Consensus guidelines from the ACCP state that patient self-management of warfarin using POC devices is suitable, depending on many factors including the fact that patients must be appropriately selected and trained. The guidelines note, however, that results from POC devices differ increasingly from laboratory INRs above the therapeutic range, and that incorrect calibration of the International Sensitivity Index of the POC instruments has been reported, among other problems. A meta-analysis of 14 randomized trials of self-monitoring with POC INR devices reported significantly fewer thromboembolic events, major hemorrhage, and all-cause mortality. Even for self-dosing based on self-monitoring, there were significantly fewer thromboembolic events and deaths, but the reduction in major hemorrhage was not significant.[33] Self-testing allows for more frequent testing. The proportion of INR results within the therapeutic range was reported in 11 studies and was significantly increased in 6 of these studies (and was nonsignificantly increased in 5 studies).[33] A randomized trial in elderly patients (>60 years old) using CoaguChek S showed reduced hemorrhage and thrombosis in the self-management group compared with usual care.[30] This type of clinical improvement is seen when self-testing is compared with management by usual care/general physician's office, but self-testing compared with a dedicated anticoagulation management service does not show such improvement.[1,34] Although not among the formal recommendations, it is suggested in the ACCP guidelines that the health care provider assess the patient and his or her device once or twice per year using duplicate testing on the patient/POC device and the physician's office equipment or laboratory.[34] Gardiner and colleagues[1] recommended that the patient's POC result should be compared with the clinic's device and the laboratory every 6 months. In addition, POC INR results between 4 and 8 should be repeated with the POC device for confirmation, and INR values greater than 8 should be confirmed by same day testing in a clinical laboratory.[1]

When validating or revalidating a POC device, the commonly used criterion to assess agreement between two methods is INR values from the device should be in the same clinical category as the result from the reference method/clinical laboratory (ie, both values should be within, above, or below the therapeutic range) or be within 0.4 INR of each other.[35,36] An alternative set of criteria requires that 85% of result pairs that are within the therapeutic range should be within 0.5 INR of each other.[1] According to the consensus document International Standards Organization 17,593:2007 criteria, when the INR is less than 2.0, more than 90% of paired INR results should be within 0.5 INR of each other; when the INR is greater than 2.0, paired results should be within 30% of each other.[31]

For patients who have a lupus anticoagulant, POC testing might not be suitable, because the lupus anticoagulant can artifactually prolong the INR with various POC devices,[37] as can also occur with some laboratory INR reagents. Chromogenic factor X assays can be performed to determine whether the POC INR is affected by the lupus anticoagulant.[37]

Coaguchek XS Plus INR values agreed well with laboratory INR values, but elevated fibrinogen apparently led to overestimation of the INR on the POC device, particularly for fibrinogen levels greater than 7 g/L (700 mg/dL).[31] In another recent study, more than 90% of CoaguChek XS and i-STAT (Abbott, Princeton, New Jersey) results and 88% of CoaguChek S results were within 0.4 INR of the reference laboratory result.[29] With CoaguChek S, 92% of result pairs were within 0.5 INR, and for Coagu-Chek XS and i-STAT, 98% of paired results were within 0.5 INR compared with the reference laboratory result.[29]

There is some evidence that the hematocrit can influence whole-blood POC INR results.[38] The manufacturer of CoaguChek XS claims that the device corrects the INR for hematocrit values that are within a specified range. The manufacturer also maintains that CoaguChek XS is not affected by therapeutic levels of heparin or low-molecular-weight heparin (LMWH). The lack of interference from heparin or LMWH is important for patients transitioning from heparin or LMWH to warfarin.

D-DIMER POINT-OF-CARE ASSAYS

D-dimer testing has been used for a variety of purposes, most commonly as part of the assessment for VTE or disseminated intravascular coagulation. More recently, D-dimer testing has been studied as a possible predictor of recurrent VTE following the discontinuation of anticoagulant therapy. Several POC D-dimer assays are available. These assays are typically rapid and are performed on whole blood or plasma, depending on the assay. Their suitability for excluding VTE is variable and they might not be sufficiently sensitive to be safely used for this purpose. A semiquantitative whole-blood erythrocyte agglutination assay (SimpliRED, AGEN Inc, Brisbane, Australia) is not sufficiently sensitive to exclude VTE in most studies, with sensitivities in the range of 56% to 94% and NPVs in the range of 52% to 97%,[39,40] but one study reported good sensitivity when used in conjunction with alveolar dead-space measurement.[41]

A rapid, whole-blood or plasma fluorescence immunoassay can deliver results in 15 minutes (Triage D-Dimer, Biosite Diagnostics, San Diego, California). One study found that it was 91% sensitive for VTE, prompting the investigators to suggest that the cutoff be reduced from 400 to 350 ng/mL to raise the sensitivity to 95% (with correspondingly lower specificity).[42] When compared with a reference method, 96% of specimens that were positive by the reference method were also positive by this POC immunoassay in citrated plasma (this particular POC test is approved for use with EDTA).[43] In comparison to another D-dimer method, the correlation coefficient was 0.96 in citrated plasma, although the coefficient of variation of the POC immunoassay was the highest among the four methods studied.[44] When implemented in an emergency department to shorten the turnaround time of D-dimer testing, it reduced length of stay in the emergency department and reduced the number of hospital admissions.[45]

A rapid, whole-blood (or plasma), solid-phase radial partition immunossay can deliver results in approximately 14 minutes (Stratus D-Dimer, Siemens Corporation). The assay involves adding the sample to a glass filter paper containing a capture antibody, followed by adding an enzyme-labeled antibody and then substrate, and measuring fluorescence.[46] It was 96.5% sensitive at 400 ng/mL but 100% sensitive at 350 ng/mL with correspondingly lower specificity.[47] In another study, a cutoff of 440 to 450 ng/mL was 95% sensitive.[46]

A rapid, immunoturbidimetric (latex agglutination) assay can generate results in 4 minutes in citrated plasma (MiniQuant, Trinity Biotech, Bray, Ireland). Because plasma specimens are used, centrifugation time is also required in addition to the 4-minute assay time. Sensitivity was 96% using a cutoff of 550 ng/mL and 100% using a cutoff of 375 ng/mL, with correspondingly less specificity at the lower cutoff.[48] A subsequent study by these investigators reported a sensitivity of 94% and an NPV of 54% using the 375 ng/mL cutoff.[49] Other studies have reported sensitivities of 96% using a cutoff of 200 ng/mL[50] and 95% using a cutoff of 250 ng/mL.[51] An additional study noted that the sensitivity was 90.4% at 334 ng/mL, but the sensitivity improved to 98.7% when combined with pretest probability, as was seen with other assays.[52]

A whole-blood dual monoclonal antibody sandwich immunoassay (Cardiac D-Dimer, Roche Diagnostics) contains two specific monoclonal anti-D-dimer antibodies, one of which is biotinylated and the other gold labeled. The reaction time is 8 minutes. When D-dimer is present in the specimen, a sandwich complex is formed with the D-dimer and the two antibodies. Streptavidin, immobilized along a stripe in the read window, binds to biotin in the complex, turning reddish purple. The color is detected optically when placed in the reader. This assay was reportedly 89% sensitive for deep venous thrombosis in one study[53] and 97% sensitive for deep venous thrombosis in another[54] at 0.5 µg/mL, and 100% sensitive at 0.4 µg/mL.[55]

ACTIVATED CLOTTING TIME POINT-OF-CARE ASSAYS

The ACT is a whole-blood clotting time that is almost always performed at the POC rather than within a clinical laboratory. It is used to monitor heparin and occasionally argatroban or other direct thrombin inhibitors, particularly at high concentrations when the PTT cannot be used, such as with cardiopulmonary bypass surgery. At high concentrations of heparin (or argatroban or other direct thrombin inhibitors), the PTT becomes unclottable. To perform this test, clotting is initiated in a blood sample by an activator of the intrinsic pathway of coagulation, and the time until clot formation is measured in seconds. There is no need for specimen transportation to the laboratory or centrifugation, and the baseline clotting time is approximately 70 to 180 seconds (depending on the method and the patient); thus, the turnaround time is very fast.

It is important to note that ACT devices from different manufacturers are not interchangeable. The reference range and the therapeutic target ACT vary considerably between instruments. In some instances, the target ACT is not well defined. Even different cartridges within the same manufacturer's device can have different reference ranges and therapeutic target ACTs, as was shown for the "low-range" and "high-range" Medtronic cartridges (ACT PLUS, Medtronic Inc, Minneapolis, Minnesota).[56] Some types of differences between analyzers have been surprising. For example, it was shown that ACT values are higher with heparin using Celite CA510 tubes on Hemo-chron 401 (International Technidyne Corporation) compared with Medtronic ACT PLUS devices.[57] Unexpectedly, with argatroban anticoagulation, the opposite pattern was seen: the ACT values were higher on the Medtronic device than with the Hemochron device.[57] Thus, when first bringing a new ACT device into clinical use, each institution needs to carefully validate its ACT target ranges.

Knowing the anti-Xa (heparin) level that corresponds to an ACT from a particular device could be useful in the initial validation of an ACT device and for subsequent troubleshooting with difficult specimens or patients. An ACT longer than 300 seconds with Hemochron 401 corresponded to an anti-Xa level greater than 1.48 IU/mL.[57] With concomitant eptifibatide in addition to heparin, the corresponding anti-Xa level for the same Hemochron ACT result appeared to be lower compared with those on heparin alone (at a Hemochron ACT of 275 seconds, the corresponding anti-Xa level with ep-tifibatide was 0.85 IU/mL; with no eptifibatide, it was 1.46 IU/mL). The variation in anti-Xa level for the same Medtronic ACT PLUS result with eptifibatide therapy was less apparent (at a Medtronic ACT of 225 seconds, the eptifibatide level was 1.93 IU/mL; with no eptifibatide, it was 1.64 IU/mL).[57]

Anti-Xa levels have also been helpful in establishing the ACT cutoff below which removal of the arterial sheath is safe after PCI.[57]

The ACT has several limitations.[58] The ACT is less precise than the PTT, and the assay does not always correlate well with the PTT or with heparin concentration (anti-Xa levels). Results are influenced by a variety of variables, including platelet count, platelet function, factor deficiencies, ambient temperature, hypothermia, hemodilution, and lupus anticoagulants. When a lupus anticoagulant is present, a heparin (anti-Xa) assay can be used to determine the level of anticoagulation. Apro-tinin prolongs celite-based ACTs but generally not kaolin-based ACTs. Thus, celite-based ACTs may overestimate the amount of heparin anticoagulation when aprotinin is present. Very high doses of aprotinin, such as following a large initial bolus, may also prolong kaolin-based ACTs. In the recent past, aprotinin was often used during coro-nary artery bypass surgery to decrease bleeding, but its use has substantially declined following some studies linking aprotinin with increased adverse outcomes.[59,60]

Some ACT devices offer "heparin management" options, which typically add substantially to the cost of the testing. Individual patients respond differently to the same dose of heparin, largely due to differences in the levels of acute-phase-reactant proteins, which are proteins that become elevated during illness, injury, stress, or postoperatively. A number of these proteins bind and neutralize heparin, such that patients who have high levels of these proteins will need higher heparin doses to achieve a target clotting time prolongation. To address this issue, before cardiopulmo-nary bypass surgery, heparin management ACT devices can perform an ACT after adding a known quantity of heparin to the specimen to determine the individual patient's responsiveness to heparin and to calculate a recommended heparin dose. At the conclusion of a cardiopulmonary bypass operation, these devices can perform an ACT after adding a known quantity of protamine to the specimen to determine how much heparin is present and to recommend a protamine dose for the patient to reverse the heparin effect. These devices have obvious theoretic advantages, but peer-reviewed published data are needed to assess their effectiveness.

SUMMARY

POC testing is available for a variety of coagulation tests, offering a rapid turnaround time. Clinicians using these devices should be aware of their limitations. Additional studies are eagerly awaited regarding potential future uses of POC coagulation testing, including the role of platelet function testing and ACT heparin management systems.

REFERENCES

1. Gardiner C, Mackie S, Mackie I. Point-of-care testing in hemostasis. In: Kitchen S, Olson J, Preston FE, editors. Quality in laboratory hemostasis and thrombosis. Hoboken (NJ): Wiley-Blackwell; 2009. p. 72–80.
2. Paniccia R, Antonucci E, Gori AM, et al. Comparison of different methods to evaluate the effect of aspirin on platelet function in high-risk patients with ischemic heart disease receiving dual antiplatelet treatment. Am J Clin Pathol 2007; 128(1):143–9.
3. Hayward CP, Harrison P, Cattaneo M, et al. Platelet function analyzer (PFA)-100 closure time in the evaluation of platelet disorders and platelet function. J Thromb Haemost 2006;4(2):312–9.
4. Schlammadinger A, Kerenyi A, Muszbek L, et al. Comparison of the O'Brien filter test and the PFA-100 platelet analyzer in the laboratory diagnosis of von Willebrand's disease. Thromb Haemost 2000;84(1):88–92.
5. Campo G, Valgimigli M, Frangione A, et al. Prognostic value of serial platelet reactivity measurements on long-term clinical outcome in patients with ST-elevation myocardial infarction undergoing primary PCI. J Thromb Haemost 2008;6(10): 1824–6.
6. Michelson AD, Cattaneo M, Eikelboom JW, et al. Aspirin resistance: position paper of the Working Group on Aspirin Resistance. J Thromb Haemost 2005; 3(6):1309–11.
7. Patrono C, Baigent C, Hirsh J, et al. Antiplatelet drugs: American College of Chest Physicians Evidence-Based Clinical Practice Guidelines (8th edition). Chest 2008;133(6 Suppl):199S–233S.
8. Douketis JD, Berger PB, Dunn AS, et al. The perioperative management of antithrombotic therapy: American College of Chest Physicians Evidence-Based Clinical Practice Guidelines (8th edition). Chest 2008;133(6 Suppl):299S–339S.
9. Campbell CL, Smyth S, Montalescot G, et al. Aspirin dose for the prevention of cardiovascular disease: a systematic review. JAMA 2007;297(18):2018–24.
10. Gum PA, Kottke-Marchant K, Welsh PA, et al. A prospective, blinded determination of the natural history of aspirin resistance among stable patients with cardiovascular disease. J Am Coll Cardiol 2003;41(6):961–5.
11. Bliden KP, DiChiara J, Tantry US, et al. Increased risk in patients with high platelet aggregation receiving chronic clopidogrel therapy undergoing percutaneous coronary intervention: is the current antiplatelet therapy adequate? J Am Coll Cardiol 2007;49(6):657–66.
12. Buonamici P, Marcucci R, Migliorini A, et al. Impact of platelet reactivity after clopidogrel administration on drug-eluting stent thrombosis. J Am Coll Cardiol 2007; 49(24):2312–7.
13. Chen WH, Cheng X, Lee PY, et al. Aspirin resistance and adverse clinical events in patients with coronary artery disease. Am J Med 2007;120(7):631–5.
14. Buch AN, Singh S, Roy P, et al. Measuring aspirin resistance, clopidogrel responsiveness, and postprocedural markers of myonecrosis in patients undergoing percutaneous coronary intervention. Am J Cardiol 2007;99(11):1518–22.
15. Price MJ, Endemann S, Gollapudi RR, et al. Prognostic significance of postclopidogrel platelet reactivity assessed by a point-of-care assay on

thrombotic events after drug-eluting stent implantation. Eur Heart J 2008; 29(8):992–1000.

16. Marcucci R, Gori AM, Paniccia R, et al. Cardiovascular death and nonfatal myocardial infarction in acute coronary syndrome patients receiving coronary stenting are predicted by residual platelet reactivity to ADP detected by a point-of-care assay: a 12-month follow-up. Circulation 2009;119(2):237–42.

17. Patti G, Nusca A, Mangiacapra F, et al. Point-of-care measurement of clopidogrel responsiveness predicts clinical outcome in patients undergoing percutaneous coronary intervention results of the ARMYDA-PRO (Antiplatelet therapy for Reduction of MYocardial Damage during Angioplasty-Platelet Reactivity predicts Outcome) study. J Am Coll Cardiol 2008;52(14):1128–33.

18. Gianetti J, Parri MS, Sbrana S, et al. Platelet activation predicts recurrent ischemic events after percutaneous coronary angioplasty: a 6 months prospective study. Thromb Res 2006;118(4):487–93.

19. Marcucci R, Paniccia R, Antonucci E, et al. Usefulness of aspirin resistance after percutaneous coronary intervention for acute myocardial infarction in predicting one-year major adverse coronary events. Am J Cardiol 2006;98(9):1156–9.

20. Andersen K, Hurlen M, Arnesen H, et al. Aspirin non-responsiveness as measured by PFA-100 in patients with coronary artery disease. Thromb Res 2002;108(1):37–42.

21. Pamukcu B, Oflaz H, Onur I, et al. Clinical relevance of aspirin resistance in patients with stable coronary artery disease: a prospective follow-up study (PROSPECTAR). Blood Coagul Fibrinolysis 2007;18(2):187–92.

22. Mega JL, Close SL, Wiviott SD, et al. Cytochrome p-450 polymorphisms and response to clopidogrel. N Engl J Med 2009;360(4):354–62.

23. Simon T, Verstuyft C, Mary-Krause M, et al. Genetic determinants of response to clopidogrel and cardiovascular events. N Engl J Med 2009;360(4):363–75.

24. Ho PM, Maddox TM, Wang L, et al. Risk of adverse outcomes associated with concomitant use of clopidogrel and proton pump inhibitors following acute coronary syndrome. JAMA 2009;301(9):937–44.

25. Juurlink DN, Gomes T, Ko DT, et al. A population-based study of the drug interaction between proton pump inhibitors and clopidogrel. CMAJ 2009;180(7): 713–8.

26. Freedman JE, Hylek EM. Clopidogrel, genetics, and drug responsiveness. N Engl J Med 2009;360(4):411–3.

27. Poller L, Keown M, Ibrahim SA, et al. Quality assessment of CoaguChek point-of-care prothrombin time monitors: comparison of the European community-approved procedure and conventional external quality assessment. Clin Chem 2006;52(10):1843–7.

28. Christensen TD, Larsen TB, Jensen C, et al. International normalised ratio (INR) measured on the CoaguChek S and XS compared with the laboratory for determination of precision and accuracy. Thromb Haemost 2009;101(3): 563–9.

29. Karon BS, McBane RD, Chaudhry R, et al. Accuracy of capillary whole blood international normalized ratio on the CoaguChek S, CoaguChek XS, and i-STAT 1 point-of-care analyzers. Am J Clin Pathol 2008;130(1):88–92.

30. Siebenhofer A, Rakovac I, Kleespies C, et al. Self-management of oral anticoagulation reduces major outcomes in the elderly. A randomized controlled trial. Thromb Haemost 2008;100(6):1089–98.

31. Deom A, Reber G, Tsakiris DA, et al. Evaluation of the CoaguChek XS Plus system in a Swiss community setting. Thromb Haemost 2009;101(5):988–90.

32. Torreiro EG, Fernandez EG, Rodriguez RM, et al. Comparative study of accuracy and clinical agreement of the CoaguChek XS portable device versus standard laboratory practice in unexperienced patients. Thromb Haemost 2009;101(5): 969–74.

33. Heneghan C, Alonso-Coello P, Garcia-Alamino JM, et al. Self-monitoring of oral anticoagulation: a systematic review and meta-analysis. Lancet 2006; 367(9508):404–11.

34. Ansell J, Hirsh J, Hylek E, et al. Pharmacology and management of the vitamin K antagonists: American College of Chest Physicians Evidence-Based Clinical Practice Guidelines (8th edition). Chest 2008;133(6 Suppl):160S–98S.

35. Anderson DR, Harrison L, Hirsh J. Evaluation of a portable prothrombin time monitor for home use by patients who require long-term oral anticoagulant therapy. Arch Intern Med 1993;153(12):1441–7.

36. van den Besselar AM. A comparison of INRs determined with a whole blood prothrombin time device and two international reference preparations for thromboplastin. Thromb Haemost 2000;84(3):410–2.

37. Perry SL, Samsa GP, Ortel TL. Point-of-care testing of the international normalized ratio in patients with antiphospholipid antibodies. Thromb Haemost 2005;94(6): 1196–202.

38. van den Besselaar AM, Witteveen E, van der Meer FJ. Influence of haematocrit on international normalised ratio (INR) differences between a whole blood point-of-care coagulation monitor and reference prothrombin time in plasma. Thromb Haemost 2008;100(6):1181–4.

39. Heim SW, Schectman JM, Siadaty MS, et al. D-dimer testing for deep venous thrombosis: a metaanalysis. Clin Chem 2004;50(7):1136–47.

40. Reber G, de Moerloose P, Coquoz C, et al. Comparison of two rapid D-dimer assays for the exclusion of venous thromboembolism. Blood Coagul Fibrinolysis 1998;9(4):387–8.

41. Kline JA, Israel EG, Michelson EA, et al. Diagnostic accuracy of a bedside D-dimer assay and alveolar dead-space measurement for rapid exclusion of pulmonary embolism: a multicenter study. JAMA 2001;285(6):761–8.

42. Ghys T, Achtergael W, Verschraegen I, et al. Diagnostic accuracy of the Triage D-dimer test for exclusion of venous thromboembolism in outpatients. Thromb Res 2008;121(6):735–41.

43. Lee-Lewandrowski E, Van Cott EM. Evaluation of the Biosite Triage® quantitative whole blood D-dimer assay and comparison with the bioMerieux VIDAS® D-dimer exclusion test: validation and utility for use in the central laboratory and at the point of care. Point of Care 2005;4:133–7.

44. La'ulu SL, Dominguez CM, Roberts WL. Performance characteristics of the AxSYM D-dimer assay. Clin Chim Acta 2008;390(1–2):148–51.

45. Lee-Lewandrowski E, Nichols J, VanCott EM, et al. Implementation of a rapid whole blood D-dimer test in the emergency department of an urban academic medical center: impact on ED length of stay and ancillary test utilization. Am J Clin Pathol, in press.

46. Freyburger G, Reboul MP, Labrouche S, et al. Diagnosis accuracy of a new challenger for thrombosis exclusion, the Stratus CS DDMR. Clin Chim Acta 2005; 354(1–2):181–9.

47. Reber G, Bounameaux H, Perrier A, et al. A new rapid point-of-care D-dimer enzyme-linked immunosorbent assay (Stratus CS D-dimer) for the exclusion of venous thromboembolism. Blood Coagul Fibrinolysis 2004;15(5):435–8.

48. Shitrit D, Heyd J, Raveh D, et al. Diagnostic value of the D-dimer test in deep vein thrombosis: improved results by a new assay method and by using discriminate levels. Thromb Res 2001;102(2):125–31.
49. Shitrit D, Levi H, Huerta M, et al. Appropriate indications for venous duplex scanning based on D-dimer assay. Ann Vasc Surg 2002;16(3):304–8.
50. Gosselin RC, Owings JT, Kehoe J, et al. Comparison of six D-dimer methods in patients suspected of deep vein thrombosis. Blood Coagul Fibrinolysis 2003; 14(6):545–50.
51. Schutgens RE, Haas FJ, Gerritsen WB, et al. The usefulness of five D-dimer assays in the exclusion of deep venous thrombosis. J Thromb Haemost 2003; 1(5):976–81.
52. Gardiner C, Pennaneac'h C, Walford C, et al. An evaluation of rapid D-dimer assays for the exclusion of deep vein thrombosis. Br J Haematol 2005;128(6): 842–8.
53. Bucek RA, Quehenberger P, Feliks I, et al. Results of a new rapid d-dimer assay (cardiac d-dimer) in the diagnosis of deep vein thrombosis. Thromb Res 2001; 103(1):17–23.
54. Dempfle CE, Korte W, Schwab M, et al. Sensitivity and specificity of a quantitative point of care D-dimer assay using heparinized whole blood, in patients with clinically suspected deep vein thrombosis. Thromb Haemost 2006;96(1):79–83.
55. Legnani C, Fariselli S, Cini M, et al. A new rapid bedside assay for quantitative testing of D-dimer (Cardiac D-Dimer) in the diagnostic work-up for deep vein thrombosis. Thromb Res 2003;111(3):149–53.
56. Arpino PA, Cronin-Jenkins S, Misiano D, et al. Comparing the activated clotting times obtained from 2 point-of-care devices in patients receiving unfractionated heparin during percutaneous coronary intervention. Point of Care 2008;7:30–3.
57. Chia S, Van Cott EM, Raffel OC, et al. Comparison of activated clotting times obtained using Hemochron and Medtronic analysers in patients receiving antithrombin therapy during cardiac catheterisation. Thromb Haemost 2009;101(3): 535–40.
58. Kratz A, Van Cott EM. Activated clotting time: methods and clinical applications. Point of Care 2005;4:90–4.
59. Mangano DT, Tudor IC, Dietzel C. The risk associated with aprotinin in cardiac surgery. N Engl J Med 2006;354(4):353–65.
60. Mangano DT, Miao Y, Vuylsteke A, et al. Mortality associated with aprotinin during 5 years following coronary artery bypass graft surgery. JAMA 2007;297(5):471–9.

Point-of-Care Testing and Molecular Diagnostics: Miniaturization Required

Frederick L. Kiechle, MD, PhD[a],*, Carol A. Holland, PhD[b]

KEYWORDS

• Point-of-care testing • Molecular diagnostics • MRSA • PCR
• Miniaturization • Amplification

Molecular diagnostic tests can be divided into two primary groups according to frequency of testing. In the first group are tests designed to detect the presence of mutations or sequences in the human genome associated with specific diseases. These tests only need to be performed once in a specific individual's lifetime. Of course, the discovery of additional disease-linked mutations may initiate additional investigation. These tests, for the most part, are considered part of the routine workload and do not require a rapid turnaround time. In the second group are molecular diagnostic assays designed to detect infectious agents,[1,2] single nucleotide polymorphisms or mutations associated with drug metabolism, or the recurrence of a mutation specifically associated with a tumor the patient has had.[3] Bacterial, viral, fungal, and parasitic infections are often life threatening, which means rapid identification is required for initiation of appropriate treatment. These types of infections include sepsis, meningitis, and hospital-associated infections, such as methicillin-resistant *Staphylococcus aureus* (MRSA). These types of infections can often be eradicated or suppressed and can recur, in which case the same molecular assay for detection would have to be repeated.[1] One example is the assay for monitoring of the amount of circulating viral particles per milliliter of blood. This is termed a viral load level and is used to monitor therapeutic efficacy and clinical course in such infections as HIV and hepatitis C virus.[4,5] Drug-metabolizing enzymes determine the extent to which an individual is able to metabolize a given drug. Individuals are classified as slow,

[a] Department of Pathology, Pathology Consultants of South Broward, LLP, Memorial Regional Hospital, 3501 Johnson Street, Hollywood, FL 33021, USA
[b] Beckman Coulter, Inc, High Sensitivity Testing Group, 200 South Kraemer Boulevard, Brea, CA 92821, USA
* Corresponding author.
E-mail address: fkiechle@mhs.net (F.L. Kiechle).

Clin Lab Med 29 (2009) 555–560
doi:10.1016/j.cll.2009.06.013
0272-2712/09/$ – see front matter © 2009 Elsevier Inc. All rights reserved.

labmed.theclinics.com

normal, or rapid metabolizers. Common drugs affected by these enzymes include antidepressants, antipsychotics, beta-blockers, and warfarin.[6] Minimal residual disease detection refers to the analysis of tissue/cells in a patient previously diagnosed with a malignancy. The analysis is needed to determine whether therapy was successful or if rare malignant cells are present. For example, monitoring JAK2 V617F mutation has been identified in the majority of Philadelphia chromosome–negative myeloproliferative disorders with minimal residual disease following specific treatment.[3] In all of these cases, the ability to perform the molecular assay at the point of care would allow the correct treatment decision to be made quickly and accurately.

Perhaps the area that will see the biggest impact with the move to molecular point-of-care testing (POCT) is that of infectious diseases. The increasing number of outbreaks of emerging novel infectious diseases[7–12] threatening human health is a result of multiple factors, including rapid pathogen mutation rates, transformation of nonhuman pathogens into human pathogens, and recombination of nonhuman pathogen with human pathogens.[13] The general dilemma is the clinical need for the identification of the pathogen in 2 to 6 hours. Most culture methods for viruses, bacteria, and fungi require a day or more for results. Identification of a bacterium by molecular methods will facilitate the initiation of therapy. However, this is based on organism identification and typical antibiotic sensitivity patterns for that organism. Generally, molecular assays cannot provide direct information related to the antibiotic sensitivity of the organism. Instead, they indirectly identify the presence or absence of resistance-carrying genes.[11,12] MRSA is an example of this generalization, where the presence of the mecA gene infers resistance to methicillin.[11] The miniaturization of the space required to extract the nucleic acid, add the reagents for polymerase chain reaction (PCR), and accommodate the thermocycler for amplification[14] could lead to the development of a molecular diagnostic device small enough to be moved from patient to patient for POCT.[15,16] This technology would be simple to use and could be employed in underdeveloped countries for rapid identification of infectious organisms.[7,14]

TYPICAL MOLECULAR ASSAY TODAY

When asked to describe a typical molecular assay, one would say there are three main processes: extraction and purification (EP) of the nucleic acid, amplification of a selected area of the nucleic acid (the "target" sequence), and detection of the amplified product (the "amplicon"). These steps form the basis for most clinical molecular assays on the market today. EP is accomplished by first lysing the cell or viral particle, releasing the nucleic acid. Standard lysis methods involve the use of chemicals, heat, sonication, or pressure. Purification involves the removal of contaminating cellular components. Nucleic acids have an affinity for silica-based particles. Several manufacturers have attached silica or similar particles to filters or magnetic beads, allowing easy separation from cellular debris, which is then washed away. The nucleic acid is subsequently eluted off the particles in a purified form. Modifications include binding small oligonucleotides (short sequences of nucleic acids) to the filters or beads, which capture nucleic acids specific for the target being isolated. The entire EP protocol takes approximately 30 minutes to complete. Several manufacturers have developed systems that automate the entire EP process.

Amplification of the purified nucleic acid is either signal or target based. Signal amplification methods, such as the branched DNA method, add multiple copies of a dye to a single copy of a target. Target amplification methods make more of the starting target nucleic acid, thus the name. They include the PCR, nucleic acid sequence-based amplification (NASBA), and transcription-mediated amplification, among others.[1,17] The amplification reaction components differ, depending on the method chosen, but normally include adding enzyme, nucleotides, cofactors, and buffers to the purified nucleic acid. The setup time for a single reaction is roughly 10 minutes. Automated reaction setup is available postextraction for some assays. Amplification protocols typically involve up to 40 "cycles," and one to three different temperatures. Average total cycle time is approximately 30 to 40 minutes.

Detection also varies by assay. Traditionally, a fluorescent intercalating dye, such as ethidium bromide, is added to the amplicon, which is then subjected to agarose gel electrophoresis. Visualization of the correct size fragment serves as identification. Other methods involving ELISA-type chemical reactions or chemiluminescence are also used. Depending on the method, the detection step can add minutes to hours to the assay. In addition, the amplicon must be removed from the reaction tube, creating potential contamination issues. The coupling of the amplification and detection steps allows the product to be identified as it is being made. Such assays are referred to as real-time assays. These assays alleviate the potential problem of contamination because they are performed in a single tube. Real-time PCR assays are currently popular for infectious-disease testing. Real-time NASBA and other real-time technologies are also being developed. The miniaturization of these real-time technologies shows the most potential for point-of-care devices.

MINIATURIZATION OF MOLECULAR ASSAYS

To achieve a portable, POCT application for molecular-based assays, the three distinct steps—nucleic acid extraction, target amplification, and detection of target(s)—need to be simplified and miniaturized.[1] In an interview with Anne Paxton[18] from *CAP Today*, Dan Farkas, PhD, the executive director of the Sequenom Center for Molecular Medicine in Grand Rapids, Michigan, stated that there are 10 or 12 companies in various stages of the development of point-of-care molecular devices. Most of these companies use microfluidics, microarrays, or small-diameter capillary tubes. At a not-so-portable size is the GeneXpert (Cepheid, Sunnyvale, California) device.[18,19] It uses a unit use device for all three of the typical molecular assay steps. Total assay time for MRSA detection on the GeneXpert is 75 minutes with total hands-on time of approximately 2 minutes.

AN IDEAL DEVICE

What feature and functions would the ideal POCT molecular device possess? Clinical applications for such a device might include rapid detection of hospital-acquired infections,[11,12] quantification of viral load,[4,5] detection of agents of bioterrorism or biowarfare,[20,21] detection of the patient's ability to metabolize a specific drug or drug class,[6] identification of the patient from whom a surgical specimen was removed,[22] and detection of minimal residual disease in a patient treated for a malignancy.[3] The primary driver for the development of this technology is faster turnaround time for the assay and subsequent result, which can be used the same day for clinical decisions related to diagnosis and treatment. The device should be handheld and, therefore, portable, and the cost per test should be less than $25. The total time to result, which includes hands-on time and analytical time, should ideally be less than half an hour for a DNA-based assay. The device should use a disposable unit use cartridge like the Cepheid GeneXpert[18,19,21] and require no preprocessing of the specimen or user intervention once the assay has been initiated. The results generated should be clear, easy to understand, and should not require any interpretation. Ideally the device would be classified under the 1988 Clinical Laboratories Improvement Amendments (CLIA) as waived.

The performance characteristics of the POCT assay should be comparable with those of the laboratory-performed version. Because miniaturization is necessary for a POCT device, some performance characteristics may suffer. One important consideration is the input volume of the starting specimen, which can affect the sensitivity, and is especially important for infectious-disease testing, where the amount of starting pathogen may be small. Accommodating larger sample volumes to maintain sensitivity is possible and can be countered by smaller elution and reaction volumes. Accuracy and precision within and among devices is another factor that requires consideration. The inclusion of external controls should help ensure comparable performance among devices. Full process controls (formerly called internal controls) that are extracted, amplified, and detected along with the target should be included in every single-use unit and will ensure that the unit is performing correctly. Because at least one process control and one target must be detected for each test, multiplexing capabilities are required.

ENABLING TECHNOLOGIES

The EP steps are perhaps the easiest and most straight forward steps to miniaturize. Currently, several manufactures have automated systems that perform the entire EP process in a single disposable unit in as little as 10 minutes. Most of these instruments are able to accommodate a variety of specimen types and volumes and to extract DNA, RNA, or total nucleic acids. For hard-to-lyse specimens, such as fresh or formalin-fixed paraffin embedded tissues, yeasts, and fungi, the inclusion of a disruption device, such as a sonic horn, as in the Cepheid GeneXpert system, will increase the potential specimen choices. Many manufacturers are using freeze-dried or lyophilized reagents for the extraction and purification process as well as amplification/detection reactions. Such reagents extend the shelf life of the reagent kits, eliminate the need for refrigeration, and are thus suitable and desirable for POCT.

Miniaturization of the thermal cycling process has been accomplished.[23] Real-time PCR assays have been successfully performed in as little as 10-μL reaction volumes. Today, several methods are used.[1,23] One employs solid phase material for conducting heat, like a metal block, and varying the temperature electronically. Another method, taking up less space, uses air to transfer heat into inexpensive standard plastic tubes, a technique that takes advantage of the time needed for the heat to reach the center of the tube. Another method, more compact still, forces a stream of air over high surface-to-volume capillary tubes containing a PCR reagent mixture. Yet another method, and the one requiring the least space, uses natural convection forces to perform thermal cycling.[23]

Microfluidic biosensors using polydimethylsiloxane microfluidics create vertical passages that generate a three-dimensional connectivity pathway, which expands the complexity of the microfluidic architecture.[24] These devices have been used to miniaturize nucleic-acid EP, nanoliter PCR, and DNA sequencing.[24] The miniaturization of conventional optical detection methods, such as absorbance, fluorescence, chemiluminescence, interferometry, and surface plasmon resonance, have successfully been applied in microfluidic biosensors.[25–27] In addition, laser-induced fluorescence methods provide good sensitivity and low detection limits for small volumes. Since DNA is not naturally fluorescent, a fluorescent intercalating dye is mixed with

DNA to generate a complex that fluoresces when excited by the appropriate wavelength.[27]

The software must be multifunctional and at a minimum be able to input user and patient identification, control the assay and system performance, perform data analysis and test interpretation, and connect to the laboratory information system. Current POCT devices contain software that performs all of these functions and provides both qualitative and quantitative results. Expanded software functionality should include multiplexing and melting curve analysis, when appropriate, for specific analytical applications.

One potential disadvantage with POCT devices is that they typically use the entire patient sample, hindering the ability to perform retesting or confirmatory testing. This also presents a problem when laboratories need to address discordant results. The POCT marketplace already contains many devices that use lateral-flow assays and electrochemical sensor detection. A small pilot project demonstrated that influenza A and B RNA trapped for 9 months on a QuickVue lateral-flow chromogenic immuno-assay (Quidel, San Diego, California) using mouse monoclonal antibody reagents could be retrieved by addition of lysis buffer and used by reverse transcriptase-PCR detection of influenza A/B RNA.[28] This study illustrates that these test strips can be saved and used for a molecular assay to evaluate discordant test results in the future.

SUMMARY

The interest in the miniaturization of the three distinct steps in PCR-based molecular methods is currently under intense investigation. Soon, portable, handheld, inexpensive POCT devices, equivalent to currently offered full-size systems, will become available to aid in the detection of mutations or in the identification of infectious agents.

REFERENCES

1. Espy MJ, Uhl JR, Sloan LM, et al. Real-time PCR in clinical microbiology: applications for routine laboratory testing. Clin Microbiol Rev 2006;19:165–256.
2. Reithinger R, Dujardin J-C. Molecular diagnosis of Leishmaniasis: current status and future applications. J Clin Microbiol 2007;45:21–5.
3. Kannim S, Thongnoppakhun W, Auewarakul CU. Two-round allele specific-polymerase chain reaction: a simple and highly sensitive method for JAK2 V617F mutation detection. Clin Chim Acta 2009;401:148–51.
4. Bain VG. Effect of HCV viral dynamics on treatment design: lessons learned from HIV. Am J Gastroenterol 2001;96:2818–28.
5. Phillips AN, Staszewski S, Weber R, et al. HIV viral load response to antiretroviral therapy according to the baseline CD4 cell count and viral load. JAMA 2001;286: 2560–7.
6. Zhu Y, Shennan M, Reynolds RR, et al. Estimation of warfarin maintenance dose based on VKORC1 (-1639G>A) and CYP2C9 genotypes. Clin Chem 2007;53: 1199–205.
7. Dong J, Olano JP, McBride JW, et al. Emerging pathogens: challenges and successes of molecular diagnostics. J Mol Diagn 2008;10:185–97.
8. Ye C, Bai X, Zhang J, et al. Spread of Streptococcus suis sequence type 7, China. Emerg Infect Dis 2008;14:787–91.
9. Zhao G-P. SARS molecular epidemiology: a Chinese fairy tale of controlling an emerging zoonotic disease in the genomics era. Philos Trans R Soc Lond B Biol Sci 2007;362:1063–81.

10. Jones KE, Patel NG, Levy MA, et al. Global trends in emerging infectious diseases. Nature 2008;451:990–3.

11. Zitterkopf NI. The advantages of molecular diagnostics in the surveillance of healthcare-associated infections. Lab Med 2008;39:623–5.

12. Calfee D, Jenkins SG. Use of active surveillance cultures to detect asymptomatic colonization with carbapenem-resistant *Klebsiella pneumoniae* in intensive care unit patients. Infect Control Hosp Epidemiol 2008;29:966–8.

13. Wolfe ND, Dunavan CP, Diamond J. Origins of major human infectious diseases. Nature 2007;447:279–83.

14. Holland CA, Kiechle FL. Point-of-care molecular diagnostic systems—past, present and future. Curr Opin Microbiol 2005;8:504–9.

15. Caliendo AM. Molecular diagnostics at POC [abstract]. Point of Care 2008;7:134.

16. Safinia L. Molecular diagnostics—point-of-care (POC) infectious disease test—bridging the gap between rapid diagnosis and treatment. Frost and Sullivan Market Insight Dec 20, 2008. Available at: http://www.frost.com/prod/servlet/market-insight-print.pag?docid=153109626. Accessed November 5, 2009.

17. Ieven M. Currently used nucleic acid amplification tests for the detection of viruses and atypicals in acute respiratory infections. J Clin Virol 2007;40:259–76.

18. Paxton A. For molecular, a brand-new way. CAP Today 2008;22(#1):35, 36, 38.

19. Kiechle FL. Point-of-care testing: 3 new developments needed for future growth. Point of Care 2008;7:97–9.

20. Zlezak T, Kuczmarski T, Oh L, et al. Comparative genomics tools applied to bio-terrorism defense. Brief Bioinform 2003;4:133–49.

21. Lim DV, Simpson JM, Kearns EA, et al. Current and developing technologies for monitoring agents of bioterrorism and biowarfare. Clin Microbiol Rev 2005;18:583–607.

22. Huijsmans R, Damen J, van der Linten H, et al. Single nucleotide polymorphism profiling assay to confirm the identity of human tissues. J Mol Diagn 2007;9:205–13.

23. Agrawal N, Ugaz VM. A buoyancy-driven compact thermocycler for rapid PCR. Clin Lab Med 2007;27:215–23.

24. Kartalov EP, Walker C, Taylor CR, et al. Microfluidic bias enable nested bio-arrays and autoregulatory devices in Newtonian fluids. Proc Natl Acad Sci U S A 2006;103:12280–4.

25. Myers FB, Lee LP. Innovations in optical microfluidic technologies for point-of-care diagnostics. Lab Chip 2008;8:2015–31.

26. Lender V. Microfluidics at the crossroad with point-of-care diagnostics. Analyst 2007;132:1186–92.

27. Shrinivasan S, Norris PM, Landers JP, et al. A low-cost, low-power consumption, miniature laser induced fluorescence system for DNA detection on a microfluidic device. Clin Lab Med 2007;27:173–81.

28. Rashid H, Hawarth E, Ellis J, et al. Reverse transcriptase-polymerase chain reaction on QuickVue influenza test strips. Point of Care 2009;8:1–3.

Point-of-Care Testing for Cardiac Markers in Acute Coronary Syndromes and Heart Failure

Kent Lewandrowski, MD

KEYWORDS

- Point-of-care • Acute coronary syndrome • Troponin
- Heart failure • B-type natriuretic peptide

Advances in technologies for performing and miniaturizing immunoassay testing have enabled the development of 15-minute whole-blood assays for various cardiac markers used in the evaluation of patients with acute coronary syndromes (ACS) and congestive heart failure. Many of the commercially available platforms have been previously described.[1,2] Available markers in point-of-care testing (POCT) formats include cardiac troponin I and T, creatine kinase isoenzyme containing M and B subunits (CK-MB), myoglobin, B-type natriuretic peptide (BNP), and N-terminal prohormone brain natriuretic peptide (NT-proBNP). Various combinations of these markers are available on small bench-top or handheld devices from a variety of manufacturers, permitting true rapid whole-blood testing in the emergency department or in hospital chest-pain units. Rapid whole-blood cardiac-marker testing devices have also proven useful in centralized stat laboratories. In many cases, the analytical and clinical performance of these assays is equivalent or nearly equal to that of conventional central laboratory testing using automated immunoassay platforms.[3] The availability of rapid high-quality point-of-care tests for patients with cardiovascular disease can facilitate restructuring of conventional approaches to patients with ACS and heart failure,[4,5] and may have the potential to improve medical outcomes.

TROPONINS, CREATINE KINASE ISOENZYME CONTAINING M AND B SUBUNITS, AND MYOGLOBIN
Clinical Considerations

Each year, approximately 8 million Americans present with nontraumatic chest pain[1] suggestive of a possible ACS. ACS encompass a range of myocardial ischemia,

Clinical Services (Anatomic and Clinical Pathology), Massachusetts General Hospital, Harvard Medical School, 55 Fruit Street, Gray 5 Chemistry, Boston, MA 02114, USA
E-mail address: klewandrowski@partners.org

Clin Lab Med 29 (2009) 561–571
doi:10.1016/j.cll.2009.06.007
labmed.theclinics.com

including unstable angina, non–Q wave acute myocardial infarction (AMI), and Q wave AMI. Electrocardiographic findings may evolve over time during an AMI. Patients who present with ST elevation indicative of ischemia on ECG usually develop a Q wave AMI (**Fig. 1**). The minority develop a non–Q wave AMI. Other patients initially show no ST elevation. Most of these are eventually diagnosed with either unstable angina or a non–ST elevation AMI (NSTEMI).[6] The distinction between unstable angina and NSTEMI is based largely on the finding of elevated cardiac markers, which highlights the importance of rapid laboratory testing in the evaluation of ACS.

In patients with a typical clinical history and diagnostic ECG findings, the diagnosis and classification of ACS may be straightforward. For others, such a diagnosis and classification may be extremely challenging. Overdiagnosis of ACS leads to unnecessary hospitalization and expensive follow-up diagnostic procedures. Approximately 50% of patients admitted for the evaluation of chest pain are eventually found not to have had an ACS[1] and less than 30% of patients admitted to a coronary care unit rule in for an AMI.[7] Consequently the majority of patients admitted for "rule out" AMI do not have a myocardial infarction. This fact has prompted various attempts to develop rapid and reliable "rule out" AMI protocols to reduce unnecessary admissions. Many hospitals have implemented chest-pain observation units to focus resources on efficient rule-out pathways. Many hospital admissions can be avoided by not admitting low-risk patients for "rule-out AMI" protocols. On the other hand, underdiagnosis of AMI will inevitably result in "missed AMI" with potentially serious morbidity or mortality. Missed AMI has been reported to be the leading cause of lawsuits stemming from events in emergency department settings.[1,5,8]

The diagnostic criteria for AMI have evolved over the past decade. In the past, the World Health Organization defined AMI as a combination of two of following three criteria[2]:

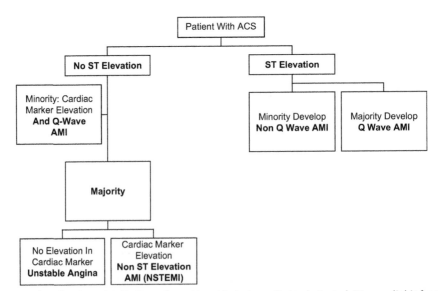

Fig. 1. Classification of ACS. (*Data from* Alpert J, Antman E, Apple F, et al. Myocardial infarction redefined. A consensus document of the joint European Society of Cardiology/American College of Cardiology Committee for the Redefinition of Myocardial Infarction. J Am Coll Cardiol 2000;36:959–69.)

Typical symptoms of ischemia
Rise and fall pattern of a cardiac marker
Typical ECG findings with the development of Q waves

In 2000, a joint consensus document from the European Society of Cardiology and the American College of Cardiology redefined AMI with a greater emphasis on the role of cardiac markers:[6]

1. Typical rise and fall of biochemical markers of myocardial necrosis (either troponin or CK-MB) with at least one of the following:
   a. Ischemic symptoms
   b. Development of pathologic Q waves on ECG
   c. ECG findings indicating ischemia (ST segment elevation or depression)
   d. Coronary artery intervention
2. Pathologic findings of an acute AMI

The ECG is highly specific for AMI when diagnostic findings are present, but the sensitivity is comparably poor (41%–75%[1]). Clinical findings may be characteristic but are unreliable for the diagnosis or exclusion of ACS in a significant percentage of patients. For these reasons, most (90%) of patients with suspected ACS require biochemical markers for diagnosis.[1] In practice, virtually all patients presenting with chest pain receive cardiac-marker testing regardless of the clinical and ECG findings. Measurement of cardiac troponin is also important for risk stratification in patients with ACS,[1] including those with unstable angina and AMI.

Most hospitals rely on established protocols involving serial cardiac markers for the evaluation of ACS. Typical protocols measure cardiac markers on admission to the emergency department, and at two time points thereafter (eg, 4–6 hours and 12–18 hours following admission). These protocols vary in timing and in the selection of individual markers. For example, at Massachusetts General Hospital, we use CK-MB and troponin on admission and then troponin at two time points thereafter. Most protocols are based on the known kinetics of cardiac-marker release associated with myocyte damage and necrosis following AMI, as shown in **Table 1**. Myoglobin is the earliest marker to rise following AMI. This marker is sensitive for myocardial necrosis and has been used by some hospitals, but is also elevated in skeletal muscle injury and therefore lacks specificity. For this reason, many hospitals do not perform myoglobin testing. CK-MB is more specific than myoglobin, but also may be elevated in skeletal muscle injury. In skeletal muscle injury, the rise in CK-MB is typically modest when compared with total CPK (percent CK-MB <5%–6% or a low CK-MB relative index). In contrast, following AMI, the rise in CK-MB relative to the total CPK is more striking,

Table 1 Kinetics of common cardiac markers in blood following AMI			
Marker	Initial Rise	Peak	Return to Baseline
Myoglobin	2–3 h[a]	6–9 h	18–24 h
CK-MB	3–8 h	10–24 h	3–4 d
Troponin	4–6 h[b]	10–24 h	Up to 7 d or more

[a] Some institutions have used a change in myoglobin (delta myoglobin) as an earlier marker. The change in myoglobin may be detected while total myoglobin values are still in the normal range (but increasing).
[b] Recent development of newer high-sensitivity troponin assays may detect an increase in troponin earlier. *Data in part from* Apple F. Acute myocardial infarction and coronary reperfusion: serum cardiac markers for the 1990s. Am J Clin Pathol 1992;97:217–26.

resulting in a higher percent CK-MB (or relative index). It is now generally agreed that cardiac troponins (either troponin I or troponin T) are the new gold standard marker for myocardial injury. Cardiac troponins are assumed to be absolutely cardiospecific and are not elevated in skeletal muscle injury or damage to other noncardiac tissues. Some hospitals have abandoned CK-MB entirely and now rely on cardiac troponin alone. This trend will likely continue.

No single cardiac-marker value can exclude or rule in the diagnosis of AMI. All cardiac markers in current use may be positive in conditions other than AMI. For example, troponin may be positive in myocarditis, cardiac contusion, and a variety of other causes. CK-MB is also elevated in these conditions and, in some patients with skeletal muscle damage, the level of CK-MB elevation may exceed the cutoff normally observed in AMI. For these reasons, in the diagnosis of AMI, it is important to observe the typical rise-and-fall pattern of cardiac markers in the context of consistent clinical findings suggestive of an ACS.

Several studies have reported accelerated "rule-out AMI" protocols using rapid serial marker testing at much shorter intervals than those used in traditional rule-out protocols.[4,5] For example, Ming and colleagues[4] reported an accelerated critical pathway for chest-pain evaluation using a combination of clinical history, ECG, and a multimarker protocol test consisting of myoglobin, CK-MB, and troponin on selected patients at 0, 30, 60, and 90 minutes from presentation to the emergency department. This approach was reported to be 100% sensitive and 94% specific for AMI. Dadkhah and colleagues[5] described a protocol using clinical and ECG findings in combination with a multimarker protocol consisting of myoglobin, CK-MB, troponin I, and BNP at admission and subsequently at 2 and 4 hours. In this study, investigators documented a reduction in patient charges, a decrease in hospital length of stay, and the elimination of unnecessary admissions to the hospital of patients with atypical chest pain. In both of these studies, rapid whole-blood point-of-care testing for cardiac markers was employed. Providing this level of speed and frequency of cardiac-marker analysis using a centralized laboratory would be extremely challenging.

Rapid turnaround time for cardiac markers is essential for rapid triage and diagnosis in patients with ACS.[4] When considering turnaround time, it is important to consider the preanalytic, analytic, and postanalytic phases of testing. In one study, the preanalytic phase constituted 42% of the total turnaround time.[9] In another study, implementation of POCT reduced the total turnaround time by 47 minutes.[10] Many other studies have demonstrated that POCT for cardiac markers can significantly reduce turnaround time.[9,11–14] Current guidelines from the American College of Cardiology–American Heart Association (ACC/AHA) recommend that total turnaround time for cardiac markers be less than 60 minutes and preferably less than 30 minutes.[15] As a result, the National Academy of Clinical Biochemistry recommends consideration of POCT for cardiac markers if the central laboratory cannot provide a reliable total turnaround time of less than 60 minutes. In some cases, these guidelines can be met using a centralized laboratory. Some laboratories have also implemented whole-blood POCT devices in the laboratory for stat testing because these devices eliminate the time needed to process plasma samples. In other hospitals, logistical problems do not permit the central laboratory to meet the recommended guidelines. In these situations, POCT may be the only practical alternative. As a result of the ACC/AHA guidelines and the obvious clinical need for rapid turnaround time, POCT for cardiac markers in the emergency department is becoming much more common.

POCT for cardiac markers using whole-blood specimens can provide rapid turnaround time with results available in as little as 15 minutes. Testing can be performed by physicians and nurses or in an emergency department satellite laboratory staffed by medical technologists.[9] The decision as to which model for performing the testing works best depends on a variety of factors. In low-volume settings, it is cost-prohibitive to staff an emergency department satellite laboratory with medical technologists unless other tests are performed to expand the menu and test volume (eg, dipstick urinalysis, urine pregnancy testing, and D-dimer). Testing performed directly by physicians and nurses is less expensive on a unit cost basis but may be difficult to manage in terms of training, ongoing competency, quality control, and regulatory compliance. Because each hospital presents unique challenges, the decision as to who will perform the testing should be made after a careful assessment of the institution's logistics and operations.

The assumption underlying POCT is that the rapid turnaround time may permit improvements in clinical outcomes or improve emergency department or hospital operations. Several studies have documented improvements in emergency department operations following implementation of cardiac-marker POCT. These improvements include a decrease in emergency department length of stay and a reduction of unnecessary hospital admissions.[14] Other studies have reported on the success of rapid rule-out protocols for ACS by employing serial cardiac-marker testing at the POCT. Presumably, these protocols reduce unnecessary admissions and emergency department length of stay because ACS can be rapidly excluded. What is clear from these studies is that each hospital presents a unique situation and that there is more than one valid approach for employing cardiac markers in the evaluation of ACS.

Despite abundant evidence that POCT for cardiac markers can reduce test turnaround time, emergency department length of stay, and unnecessary admissions, there are little published data to document improved patient outcomes, such as reductions in morbidity and mortality.[14] In a meta-analysis review of POCT cardiac-marker testing by Storrow[14] including 167 publications, only 13 articles met the study inclusion criteria of addressing one of the primary endpoints. Most of the other 153 studies reported only on the analytical performance of the point-of-care tests. The investigator concluded that "as yet there is no evidence that implementing point of care testing for cardiac biomarkers has an effect on clinical outcomes for patients being evaluated for ACS." Until new research emerges concerning the potential clinical benefits from cardiac-marker POCT, the major "evidence-based" factor supporting this testing rests on the demonstrated benefits to emergency department and hospital operations.

Analytical Considerations

Various manufacturers provide a number of options for performing whole-blood cardiac-marker testing (**Table 2**). Individual companies will not be mentioned to avoid the appearance of endorsement of a specific product. The analytical principles behind many of these products have been described in detail elsewhere[1,2] and will not be discussed further here. Each institution must determine platform and the menu of tests to offer according to accepted practice standards and local preferences. For example, some institutions use myoglobin as an early marker of AMI. Other hospitals do not include this test in the ACS panel. Hospitals that use troponin T or I in the central laboratory may find it unacceptable to use a different troponin at the point of care. For the above reasons, the laboratory should consult with emergency department physicians and cardiologists to determine the most appropriate POCT strategy for their unique situation. Often more than one approach is valid for addressing problems in clinical medicine. The evaluation of patients with suspected ACS is no exception. Regardless of the menu selected, the methods need to be validated and crossed over to tests available in the central laboratory. In many cases, this is not straightforward. For

Table 2
Options for performing whole-blood cardiac-marker testing

Option	Comments
Qualitative tests	Provides a negative or positive result; may be visually read or accompanied by a reader device; visually read tests may suffer from subjectivity and intraobserver variation; cutoff values are defined by the vendor and cannot be adjusted by the laboratory.
Quantitative tests	Marker values are determined by an instrument; cutoff values can be adjusted by the individual laboratory; values may not match those for the same marker when performed on different instruments in the central laboratory.
Discrete testing	Visually read or instrumented tests for one marker at a time; allows selection of individual tests but performing more than one test on a single sample may be time consuming.
Panel testing	Multiple markers available as a single panel; very efficient when multiple tests are required on a single specimen but may include markers that are not desired by the individual site; cost of manufacturing tends to be higher as is the cost of the panel compared with discrete testing for a single marker.
Multimarker platforms	Capable of performing a menu of tests beyond cardiac markers for ACS (eg, natriuretic peptides, d-dimer, human chorionic gonadotropin, electrolytes, drugs of abuse)

example, whole-blood samples for validation of cardiac markers may be difficult to obtain without drawing an extra tube from patients. This requires informed consent. Whole-blood values may differ from results obtained on plasma samples even on the same instrument.[16] Finally, the calibration and cutoff values used on the POCT device frequently differ from those used in the central laboratory. For example, at Massachusetts General Hospital, we perform whole-blood testing for CK-MB and troponin I in the emergency department and use a different CK-MB and troponin T in the central laboratory, as shown in **Table 3**. Because we use two different troponins and two CK-MB assays with different cutoff values, we needed to develop a strategy to reconcile results from the emergency department and the central laboratory as shown in **Fig. 2**. In the emergency department, we perform whole-blood testing and report the results as either negative, borderline, or positive. For specimens with borderline or positive results, we reflex the specimen to the central laboratory for quantitative testing. This approach also permits consistency when serial marker studies are performed in the central laboratory to document the typical rise-and-fall pattern consistent with AMI.

Decisions concerning the determination of cutoff values for cardiac troponin (and CK-MB) have received considerable attention.[15] Current guidelines recommend establishing the upper limit of normal at the 99th percentile of the reference population. At this value, the desirable imprecision of the troponin assay is recommended to be coefficient of variation of 10% or less.[15] For some POCT assays, these data are not readily available. In other cases, the analytical performance of the assays does not meet the recommended guidelines. Manufacturers will continue to improve the performance of their assays and eventually most will likely comply with these recommendations.

Technologies for performing immunoassays have made major improvements over recent years. As a result, manufacturers have introduced progressively more sensitive

Table 3
Point-of-care cardiac-marker result reporting criteria compared to central laboratory criteria at Massachusetts General Hospital in 2009

Marker	Central Laboratory	Point of Care
Troponin	Troponin T: <0.3 ng/mL, negative; 0.3–0.9 ng/mL, suggestive of myocardial necrosis; >0.9 ng/mL, indicative of myocardial necrosis	Troponin I: <0.4 ng/mL, negative; 0.4–0.7 ng/mL, borderline; >0.7 ng/mL, positive
CK-MB	<7.0 ng/mL, negative; relative index ≤3.5%	<7.5 ng/mL, negative; 7.5–15 ng/mL, borderline; >15 ng/mL, positive
Total creatine kinase	Male, 60–400 U/L; female, 40–150 U/L	Not available
Myoglobin	Not performed	Performed, not reported

assays for troponin I and T. These so-called "high-sensitivity assays" can reliably detect much lower amounts of troponin in blood than was previously possible. Troponin values that used to fall below the detection limit of the available assays can now be measured and distinguished from the 99th percentile of the normal range. It is generally viewed that these values are clinically significant, reflecting myocardial injury that was previously biochemically undetectable. As a consequence, more patients presenting with chest pain are being diagnosed with AMI.[17,18] Furthermore, it may be possible to diagnose AMI using rapid serial testing to document a change in troponin (delta troponin) using values below the absolute cutoff for AMI but nonetheless rising.[18] To a certain extent, the technologies for measuring troponins are outstripping the ability of clinicians to fully appreciate the significance of the values produced by some of these high-sensitivity assays. More research will be needed to fully appreciate the significance of small amounts of troponin in different medical

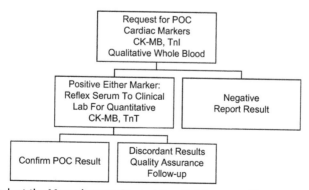

Fig. 2. Approach at the Massachusetts General Hospital for reconciling point-of-care cardiac markers with those from the central laboratory. (*Data from* Alpert J, Antman E, Apple F, et al. Myocardial infarction redefined. POC, point of care; TnI, troponin I; TnT, troponin T. A consensus document of the joint European Society of Cardiology/American College of Cardiology Committee for the Redefinition of Myocardial Infarction. J Am Coll Cardiol 2000;36:959–69; with permission.)

settings. It is also likely that some assumptions based on older studies in the literature will be reevaluated in light of new findings using improved biomarker assays.

A number of new markers that may be useful in the evaluation of patients with coronary artery disease have been described. These include markers of ischemia, inflammation, and plaque stability or rupture.[19–21] Examples include markers for ischemia-modified albumin, C-reactive protein, myeloperoxidase, soluble CD40 ligand, and fatty-acid binding protein. As yet none of these markers can be found in mainstream clinical practice nor are any assays available in formats suitable for POCT. Further research and assay development will be required to fully define what role these markers may play in the evaluation of ACS in the future.

B-TYPE NATRIURETIC PEPTIDES

Patients with congestive heart failure typically present with dyspnea or other nonspecific signs and symptoms. Approximately 5 million Americans are affected by chronic heart failure, resulting in about 1 million hospital admissions per year. Decompensated heart failure is recognized as the most common cause of hospital admission in the elderly population.[22] The severity of heart failure is usually categorized according to the New York Heart Association classification system, which divides heart failure into four grades (I–IV) based on the clinical presentation and the degree of left ventricular dysfunction. Although some cases of heart failure are easy to recognize based on clinical findings, in many patients the diagnosis can be challenging even for experienced cardiologists. Left ventricular dysfunction can be evaluated using cardiac ultrasound, but this technology is expensive, requires expert interpretation, and may not always be readily available. The discovery of the blood biomarkers BNP peptide and its N-terminal fragment NT-proBNP provided clinicians with a new laboratory approach to the diagnosis of heart failure.

BNP is synthesized in the myocardium in the form of a precursor protein that is subsequently cleaved to form proBNP and stored in granules within the myocytes. Following release into the blood, the proBNP is again cleaved into the active hormone BNP and an inactive N-terminal fragment, NT-proBNP. Unlike troponin and CK-MB, which leak from damaged myocytes, BNP functions as a neurohormone, producing diuretic, natriuretic, and vasodilatory effects. In clinical practice, measurement of both BNP and NT-proBNP have been shown to be useful in the following settings:[22–25]

> Differential diagnosis of dyspnea: Studies have shown that BNP testing is informative in the differential diagnosis of patients with acute dyspnea. These patients may have acute heart failure or other conditions, such as chronic obstructive pulmonary disease exacerbation, asthma, or pneumonia.
> Diagnosis and prognostic assessment of heart failure: Use of BNP testing has been shown to be better than clinical judgment alone in the diagnosis of mild to moderate acute heart failure. The level of blood BNP correlates with the severity of heart failure as defined by the New York Heart Association classification. Also, the higher the level of BNP, the worse the prognosis.
> As an aid in prognostic assessment of patients with ACS: Patients with ACS, including AMI, may exhibit elevations of blood levels of BNP. Elevated levels are associated with a worse prognosis and reflect significant myocardial injury, resulting in impaired left ventricular function.

Additional but still controversial potential applications for these biomarkers include use of serial marker levels to guide therapy of patients during hospitalization with acute heart failure and the use of periodic measurements to manage patients with chronic heart failure in the outpatient setting. Presumably, outpatient monitoring of patients with chronic heart failure would permit physicians to adjust therapy and potentially avoid hospitalizations due to decompensated heart failure.

A number of studies have documented that implementation of testing for BNP or NT-proBNP can result in improvements in outcomes, including improved accuracy of diagnosis,[23] decreased hospital length of stay,[24,26,27] decreased cost,[24,28] and reductions in hospital admissions for acute heart failure.[29] However, there are relatively little data to indicate that testing for these biomarkers has any measureable effect on long-term mortality.[28]

Point-of-care assays for both BNP and NT-proBNP are available from a number of commercial vendors. In fact, the first such assay was originally launched on a POCT platform before a traditional central laboratory assay was available. At present, there are no consistent data to suggest a preference for either BNP or NT-proBNP, as both appear equally accurate and clinically useful.[25] Point-of-care assays permit rapid whole-blood measurements to be determined in acute care settings, such as emergency rooms, and in outpatient settings. Although a number of studies have used point-of-care BNP assays to demonstrate improved clinical diagnosis and economic outcomes in various settings,[24,26,27] no data are yet available to demonstrate that POCT per se, as opposed to centralized testing, is uniquely able to produce these benefits. For this reason, a recommendation to support point-of-care BNP testing in preference to central laboratory testing cannot be made based on available evidence. The decision to employ POCT for this marker must therefore rely on factors related to the individual institution.

If POCT is employed in the emergency department for natriuretic peptides, the test will also need to be implemented in the central laboratory to accommodate inpatients and to support outpatient testing. This requirement raises issues concerning the potential use of two different assays in two locations, each using a different normal range and producing different values on the same patient. These issues are largely eliminated with the use of NT-proBNP because all of the existing assays are standardized to a single "parent" method. In contrast, BNP assays from different vendors produce different results and this will need to be reconciled if POCT and the central laboratory employ a different method.

SUMMARY

Advances in technologies for immunoassay testing have enabled the development of 15-minute whole-blood assays for cardiac markers used in the evaluation of patients with ACS and congestive heart failure. In many cases, the analytical performance of these assays is equivalent to testing in the central laboratory. Rapid whole-blood point-of-care assays for troponin, CK-MB, myoglobin, and BNP have facilitated efforts to restructure conventional approaches to ACS and heart failure in the emergency room.

Improvements in outcomes, including decreased emergency room and hospital length-of-stay, decreased overall cost, and earlier discharge of low-risk patients, have been documented following implementation of these technologies.

REFERENCES

1. Collinson P. Testing for cardiac markers at the point of care. Clin Lab Med 2001; 21:351–62.
2. Wu A. Point of care testing for cardiac markers: has the time come. Point of Care 2002;1:39–61.

3. Blomkalns A. Point of care testing for ACS in the emergency department. Emergency Medicine Cardiac Research and Education Group monograph. In: Blomkalns A, Gibler B, editors. American College of Emergency Physicians Scientific Assembly Satellite Symposium. Chicago IL: College of American Pathologists; 2005. Available at: www.emcreg.org.

4. Ming S, Padma K, Morissey R, et al. Ninety minute accelerated critical pathway for chest pain evaluation. Am J Cardiol 2001;88:611–6.

5. Dadkhah S, Sharain K, Sharain R, et al. The value of bedside cardiac multimarker assay in rapid and accurate diagnosis of acute coronary syndromes. Crit Pathw Cardiol 2007;6:76–84.

6. Alpert J, Antman E, Apple F, et al. Myocardial infarction redefined. A consensus document of the joint European Society of Cardiology/American College of Cardiology Committee for the redefinition of myocardial infarction. J Am Coll Cardiol 2000;36:959–69.

7. Puleo P, Meyer D, Wathen C, et al. Use of a rapid assay of subforms of creatinine kinase MB to diagnose or rule out acute myocardial infarction. N Engl J Med 1994;331:561–6.

8. Hamm C. Cardiac biomarkers for rapid evaluation of chest pain. Circulation 2001; 104:1454–9.

9. Lee-Lewandrowski E, Corboy D, Lewandrowski K, et al. Implementation of a point of care satellite laboratory in the emergency department of an academic medical center. Impact on test turnaround time and patient emergency department length of stay. Arch Pathol Lab Med 2003;127:456–60.

10. McCord J, Nowak R, McCullough P, et al. Ninety minute exclusion of acute myocardial infarction by use of quantitative point-of-care testing of myoglobin and troponin I (CHECKMATE) study. Circulation 2001;103:1832–7.

11. Di Serio F, Antonelli G, Trerotoli P, et al. Appropriateness of point of care testing (POCT) in an emergency department. Clin Chim Acta 2003;333:185–9.

12. Apple F, Chung A, Kogut M, et al. Decreased patient charges following implementation of point of care cardiac troponin monitoring in acute coronary syndrome patients in a community hospital cardiology unit. Clin Chim Acta 2006;370:191–5.

13. Ryan R, Linsell C, Hollander J, et al. A multicenter randomized controlled trial comparing central laboratory and point of care cardiac marker testing strategies: the disposition impacted by serial point of care markers in acute coronary syndromes (DISPO-ACS) trial. Ann Emerg Med 2008 [epublication ahead of print].

14. Storrow A. A systematic review of emergency department point-of-care cardiac markers and ED efficiency measures. Point of Care, in press.

15. Apple F, Jesse R, Newby K, et al. National Academy of Clinical Biochemistry and IFCC Committee for Standardization of Markers of Cardiac Damage Laboratory Medicine Practice Guidelines: analytical issues for biochemical markers of acute coronary syndromes. Clin Chem 2007;53:547–51.

16. Lee-Lewandrowski E, Benzer T, Corboy D, et al. Cardiac marker testing as part of an emergency department point-of-care satellite laboratory in a large academic medical center. Practical issues concerning implementation. Point of Care 2002; 1:145–54.

17. Casals G, Filella X, Auge J, et al. Impact of ultrasensitive cardiac troponin I dynamic changes in the new universal definition of myocardial infarction. Am J Clin Pathol 2008;130:964–98.

18. Lusky K. Troponin: new tool in an old friend. CAP Today 2009;23:1–17.

19. Morrow D, deLemos J, Sabatine M, et al. The search for a biomarker of ischemia. Clin Chem 2003;49:537–9 [editorial].
20. Apple F, Wu A, Mair J, et al. Future biomarkers of ischemia and risk stratification in acute coronary syndrome. Clin Chem 2005;51:810–24.
21. Maisel A, Bhalla V, Braunwald E. Cardiac biomarkers: a contemporary status report. Nat Clin Pract Cardiovasc Med 2006;3:24–34.
22. deFilippi C. Natriuretic peptides for diagnosing heart failure and beyond: what we know in 2007. Medscape continuing medical education 2007 (May). Available at: www.medscape.com. Accessed May 24, 2007.
23. Januzzi J, Camargo C, Anwaruddin S, et al. The N-terminal pro-BNP investigation of dyspnea in the emergency department (PRIDE) study. Am J Cardiol 2005;95: 948–54.
24. Mueller C, Scholer A, Iaule K, et al. Use of B-type natriuretic peptide in the evaluation and management of acute dyspnea. N Engl J Med 2004;350:647–54.
25. Clerico A, Fontana M, Passino C, et al. Comparison of the diagnostic accuracy of brain natriuretic peptide (BNP) and the N-terminal part of the propeptide of BNP immunoassays in chronic and acute heart failure. Clin Chem 2007;53:813–22.
26. Green S, Redmond K, Januzzi J, et al. The impact of amino-terminal pro-brain natriuretic peptide testing on hospital length of stay and morbidity in patients with acute heart failure. Arch Pathol Lab Med 2007;131:473–6.
27. Blick K. Economics of point-of-care testing for cardiac markers and B-natriuretic peptide (BNP). Point of Care 2005;4:11–4.
28. Breidthardt T, Laule K, Strohmeyer A, et al. Medical and economic long term effects of B-type natriuretic peptide testing in patients with acute dyspnea. Clin Chem 2007;53:1415–22.
29. Jourdain P, Jondeau G, Funck F, et al. Plasma brain natriuretic peptide-guided therapy to improve outcome in heart failure: the STARS-BNP Multicenter Study. J Am Coll Cardiol 2007;49:1733–9.

Provider-performed Microscopy

Frederick L. Kiechle, MD, PhD[a,b,c,*], Isabel Gauss, MT(ASCP)[a,b,c]

KEYWORDS

- Point-of-care testing • Provider-performed microscopy
- Fecal leukocytes • Fern test • Seminal fluid

Point-of-care testing (POCT) is defined as analytic testing performed outside the central laboratory using a device or devices that can be easily transported to the vicinity of the patient.[1] Chemical analysis at the patient bedside or in ward side rooms was described in London, England, in 1883.[2,3] This definition emphasizes the semiquantitative or quantitative nature of the data obtained. This emphasis is consistent with physiologic parameters, such as temperature, respiratory rate, or blood pressure, that are determined by health care professionals at the bedside or by using computer-interfaced devices. Errors in the examination of hypertensive patients made when using the indirect method of blood pressure measurement (cuff and sphygmomanometer) can be attributable to technique, equipment used, and random variability.[4–6] Training testers to follow published guidelines improved performance.[4] These findings emphasize the need for teamwork[7,8] and knowledge of published guidelines[7–12] to improve the quality of testing at the bedside. Some procedures at the bedside, however, require the evaluation of color, odor, consistency, or a semiqualitative reagent strip reaction.[13,14] For example, the location of a nasogastric tube may be evaluated by observing the color and pH of the aspirated contents.[14] Not all bedside testing results in a numerical endpoint.

Rules and regulations related to POCT are undergoing evolution, and changes should be anticipated. In general, federal law, as described by the Health Care Financing Administration in the Clinical Laboratory Improvement Amendments of 1998 (CLIA), provides the framework for most POCT standards and guidelines.[7,10] These federal regulations, using well-defined criteria, classify laboratory procedures based on their test complexity: waived, moderately complex, highly complex, and provider-performed microscopy (PPM). Certificates are issued by the Health Care Financing Administration depending on the complexity of the tests performed at the testing site (**Table 1**). **Table 2** reviews the types of laboratories enrolled in the CLIA program.

This article originally appeared in Clinics in Laboratory Medicine 2001;21(2)375–87.

[a] Department of Clinical Pathology, William Beaumont Hospital, 3601 West, 13 Mile Road, Royal Oak, MI 48073-6769, USA

[b] Beaumont Reference Laboratory, William Beaumont Hospital, Royal Oak, MI, USA

[c] Department of Pathology, Wayne State University, Detroit, MI, USA

* Corresponding author. Department of Clinical Pathology, William Beaumont Hospital, 3601 West, 13 Mile Road, Royal Oak, MI 48073-6769.

E-mail address: fkiechle@beaumont.edu (F.L. Kiechle).

Table 1 CLIA number categories	
Categories	Certificates (Biannual Fees)
1	Certificate of moderate complexity, volume-dependent ($150–$7,940)
2	CLIA waiver certificate for tests, granted status under HCFA ($150, waived)
3	CLIA certificate for provider-performed microscopy procedures ($200)

Health Care Financing Administration data from July 1999.
Abbreviation: HCFA, Health Care Financing Administration.

Bright-field or phase-contrast microscopy of labile specimens has traditionally been performed by the patient's physician at or near the point of care. Because specimen lability could compromise test accuracy, a unique regulatory approach for this testing was defined in the *Federal Register* of April 25, 1995, and revised on October 1, 1998. The following summary covers the criteria for PPM procedures:

1. The examination must be personally performed by a practitioner.
2. The procedure must be categorized as moderately complex.
3. The primary instrument for performing the test is the microscope, limited to bright-field or phase-contrast microscopy.
4. The specimen is labile or delay in performing the test could compromise the accuracy of the test result.
5. Control materials are not available to monitor the entire testing process.
6. Limited specimen handling or processing is required.

PPM procedures are performed using specimens that include body fluids and skin scrapings. The following list includes the procedures in this category[15] as of July, 1998:

1. Wet mounts, including preparation of vaginal, cervical, or skin specimens (Q0111)
2. All potassium hydroxide preparations (Q0112)
3. Pinworm examinations (Q0113)
4. Fern test (Q0114)
5. Postcoital direct, qualitative examinations of vaginal or cervical mucus (Q0015)
6. Urine sediment examinations (CPT-4 81015; for urinalysis with microscopy, use 81000, or for urinalysis performed using an automated dipstick urinalysis instrument, approved as waived, use 81001.)

Table 2 CLIA registration		
Laboratory Characteristics	No. of Laboratories	No. of Laboratories in Physician Offices
Total laboratories in nonexempt states	162,044	93,872
Total laboratories in CLIA-exempt states (New York, Oregon, Washington)	7,514	—
Application type		
Compliance (HCFA surveys)	26,045 (16%)	17,703 (19%)
Waiver	84,217 (53%)	39,633 (42%)
PPM	34,782 (21%)	29,501 (31%)
Accreditation	17,000 (10%)	7,030 (8%)

Health Care Financing Administration data from July 1999.
Abbreviation: HCFA, Health Care Financing Administration.

7. Nasal smears for granulocytes (89190)
8. Fecal leukocyte examinations (G0026)
9. Qualitative semen analysis (limited to the presence or absence of sperm and detection of motility) (G0027)

If a physician, dentist, midlevel practitioner, or physician assistant (under the supervision of a physician or in an independent practice authorized by the state) personally performs these tests on patients of his or her medical practice (including a group practice of which the physician is a member), the laboratory may receive a certificate for PPM procedures. With this certificate, the laboratory is also permitted to conduct waived tests.

EXAMPLES OF PROVIDER-PERFORMED MICROSCOPY PROCEDURES
Fecal Leukocytes

The color and consistency of stool are important aspects of initial point-of-care evaluation. Silver stools are associated with carcinoma involving the ampulla of Vater.[16] Loose, watery stools that are observed in patients who have diarrhea may be evaluated by using bacterial culture, investigating for ova, and checking for parasites and fecal leukocytes.[17] The fecal leukocyte investigation is categorized as PPM. A fleck of stool or mucus is placed on a glass slide and stained using Wright'sor Loffler methylene blue.[18] After placing a coverslip over the mixture, a rough quantitative count of mononuclear and polymorphonuclear cells is distinguished among 200 total cells. The presence of fecal leukocytes indicates the presence of an inflammatory condition caused by either a specific organism (eg, *Salmonella, Shigella*, invasive *Escherichia coli, Yersinia*, or *Entamoeba histolytica*) or nonspecific etiology (eg, ulcerative colitis or antibiotic-associated colitis).[17–19]

Fern Test

After premature rupture of the fetal membranes, the detection of amniotic fluid may be required. The protein and glucose pads on a urine dipstick may be used to rapidly distinguish amniotic fluid from maternal urine.[20] Amniotic fluid will give a positive reaction for both analytes, whereas urine will be negative unless there is maternal diabetes mellitus. Protein and pH levels may also be evaluated using a urine dipstick. Amniotic fluid is neutral or alkaline, whereas urine is usually acidic.[21] The evaluation of amniotic fluid pH and amniotic fluid crystallization (ferning) has been used to detect amniotic fluid after premature rupture of the fetal membranes.[22–24] Litmus paper, bromthymol blue, and nitrazine paper (phenaphthazine, Bristol-Myers Squibb, Princeton, New Jersey) have been used for pH determination. Nitrazine paper is still used and has a narrow pH range for color change from pH 6.4 to 6.8. Alkaline amniotic fluid will generate a blue color when its sensitivity and specificity are greater than 95%.[23,24] False-positive results may occur in the presence of blood, soaps, or infection.[23,24] The microscopic detection of amniotic fluid crystallization and the fern test are classified as PPM. Amniotic fluid after 20 weeks' gestation crystallizes on drying (**Fig. 1**),[23] whereas urine does not (**Fig. 2**). Estrogen promotes this phenomenon, and progesterone inhibits it. Slide arborization occurs in other tissues, such as serum, cerebrospinal fluid, and saliva.[23,24] The fern test has a similar sensitivity for detecting amniotic fluid in vaginal secretions, but is more specific than nitrazine paper.[23,25,26] The presence of blood at a dilution of less than 1:1 and meconium do not interfere with the fern test.[23,24] The use of a microscopic-slide fern test using saliva to determine ovulation in fertile women was found to be unreliable.[27]

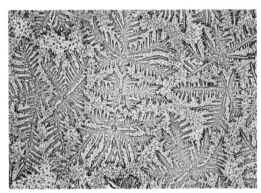

Fig. 1. Amniotic fluid dried on a slide, illustrating a positive fern test with an arborization pattern (bright field, original magnification 10).

Seminal Fluid

Seminal fluid, or semen, consists of products from various male reproductive organs: seminal vesicles (60% by volume); prostate (20%); and epididymis, vas deferens, bulbourethral glands, and urethral glands (10 to 15%).[28,29] Spermatozoa are maintained in seminal fluid. Semen analysis may be performed for a variety of reasons that dictate the complexity of the analysis required, including evaluating infertile couples,[30] detecting sexual assault,[31] verifying vasectomy effectiveness, and determining the semen's suitability for use in artificial insemination procedures.[32,33]

Semen should be collected by masturbation after a minimum of 48 hours, but not longer than 7 days, of sexual abstinence. The viscous, yellow-gray semen forms a coagulum in which the sperm are trapped. Liquefaction begins within 10 to 20 minutes and is complete within 1 hour.[28,29] Laboratory evaluation should be performed within 1.5 and 2 hours after collection. Postvasectomy patients should provide several semen specimens to assure that no viable or nonviable sperm are present. Qualitative semen analysis (limited to the presence or absence of sperm and detection of motility) is classified as PPM. A wet-mount preparation on a glass slide with a cover slip is adequate. In the emergency center, a saline wet mount from a swab of a specimen that was obtained from a sexual assault victim may be used for a point-of-care search under a microscope for motile or nonmotile sperm.[31]

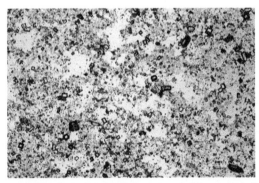

Fig. 2. Urine dried on a slide, illustrating debris and crystal formation (bright field, original magnification ×10).

Semen analysis for evaluation of a possibly infertile couple and adequacy for artificial insemination procedures requires additional procedures, including viability studies and determinations of viscosity, volume, pH, sperm concentration or count, sperm mobility, and sperm morphology.[28,29,32,34–36] Reproductive laboratories that use assisted reproductive technology are accredited on a voluntary basis by a program called the Reproductive Laboratory Accreditation Program, which was started in 1992.[32,37,38] This program is a joint venture of the College of American Pathologists and the American Society for Reproductive Medicine. Approximately 36% of these laboratories have been accredited.[38]

Pinworm Examination

Enterobius vermicularis (pinworm) is the most common nematode found in humans. The name "pinworm" is derived from the anatomic features of the tail of the worm, which is long, thin, and pointed.[39] It is most prevalent in temperate climates, and infections are most common in school-aged children.[40] Transmission is by the fecal-oral route.[41] The most frequent symptom associated with enterobiasis is pruritus ani, which occurs primarily during the evening hours, when the host is relaxed. The gravid female worm migrates from the cecum to the perianal and perineal area to deposit thousands of eggs (**Fig. 3**). Other clinical manifestations result from the migration of the gravid female worm to distal sites. For example, migration to the urogenital tract may result in recurrent urinary tract infections in young female patients.[40] Although rare, enterobiasis has also been associated with granulomas and abscesses along the distal migration track (**Fig. 4**).[42] Children suffering from enterobiasis are often nervous, restless, and irritable, and may suffer from loss of appetite, nightmares, insomnia, weight loss, and perianal pain.[39,43]

Identification of pinworms may be made either in a physician's office or in a laboratory setting. The cellulose tape method is one common methodology used by physicians. A tongue depressor or wooden applicator is covered at one end with cellophane tape. This tape-stick ensemble is pressed against the perianal region. The tape is then reversed and placed on a slide for bright-field microscopic examination. A drop of xylene or toluene may be used to dissolve the tape adhesive.[43] The specimen should be obtained just after the child awakens or at least before bathing in the morning. The physician then examines the slide for the presence of *Enterobius vermicularis* eggs, which are approximately 50 to 60 m long and have a characteristic flat side (see **Fig. 3**). Another option for detection of pinworms is a visual examination of the anal

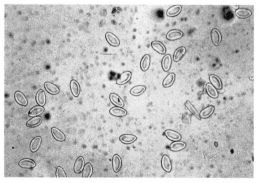

Fig. 3. Scotch-tape preparation, demonstrating the presence of *Enterobius vermicularis* eggs (bright field, original magnification ×10).

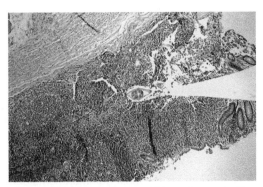

Fig. 4. Cross-section of appendix from a 4-year-old boy, demonstrating the presence of an adult *Enterobius vermicularis* worm, with prominent lateral alae and marked inflammatory reaction (hematoxylin-eosin, original magnification ×4).

area when the child is asleep. Using a flashlight, the female worm may be observed attempting to lay her eggs.[39]

Laboratory evaluation is also an option. For specimen collection, the SWUBE (Becton-Dickinson and Company, New Jersey) is available. This product includes a clear, plastic, 17-100-mm tube. The tube cap has a clear paddle attached to it that contains a sticky substance to capture the eggs. The paddle is then examined under a microscope for the presence or absence of pinworm eggs.

The traditional treatment for pinworm infection consists of a single oral dose of mebendazole. This treatment may be repeated in 2 weeks to prevent reinfection. There is also an over-the-counter product available for treating pinworm, pyrantel pamoate (Reese Pharmaceutical Co, Inc, Cleveland, Ohio).[39] The most important factor in the prevention of ringworm infection is good hygiene, including efficient hand washing.

Urine Sediment Examination

Urinalysis is defined as the physical, microscopic, or chemical examination of urine. A urine specimen has been described as a liquid tissue biopsy of the urinary tract.[15,44] There are many different factors that must be considered when performing a complete urinalysis, and this discussion will be limited to several microscopic findings. Proper specimen collection is the key to obtaining the most accurate laboratory data. The presence of a large number of squamous epithelial cells in conjunction with the presence of bacteria suggests that a sample is contaminated.

For microscopic examination of urine, 12 mL of well-mixed, fresh urine should be spun at 400 g for 5 minutes. The supernatant should be decanted and the sediment resuspended. A drop of the resuspended sediment should be placed on a glass slide with a coverslip. This should set for 30 to 60 seconds to allow for the cellular elements to settle.[15] However, centrifugation removes proteins and lipids from urine and may influence crystallization activity, especially crystal formation in vitro in processed urine.[45]

In a doctor's office setting, hematuria and pyuria are commonly evaluated microscopically in urinary sediment (**Table 3**). Hematuria is the abnormal presence of blood (red cells) in the urine. This finding may be symptomatic of many renal diseases and diseases of the genitourinary tract. Pyuria (the abnormal presence of white cells) can be indicative of infection (**Fig. 5**), but is it is not as reliable an indicator as the detection of bacteriuria using a gram stain or a culture from a fresh, midstream specimen.[44,46]

Table 3
Common causes of hematuria and pyuria

Disease	Symptoms	Cause
Hematuria renal/ genitourinary tract disease	Bleeding disorders/anticoagulation therapy Drugs (eg, cyclophosphamide)	Excessive exercise
Pyuria contamination	Bladder tumors Infection Rupture of renal or urinary tract abscess	Calculous disease

During the microscopic examination of urine, casts are also noted, if present. Casts are translucent and are composed of mucoprotein in the tubules of nephrons. There are different classifications of types of casts, based on the cast matrix, inclusions, pigments, and cells present. Examples of cast types include casts that are hyaline, waxy, and cellular. Although casts can be seen using bright-field examination, the use of phase-contrast microscopy is preferred. Large numbers of hyaline casts may be seen after strenuous exercise, but may also be indicative of renal disease.

The presence of bacteria, renal tubular cells, *Trichomonas*, crystals, yeast, or mucus should also be noted. Standardization, technical competence, and continuing education must be ensured for accurate assessment of patient samples.[44,47] A well-maintained procedure manual may assist with this task.[47]

COORDINATION OF PROVIDER-PERFORMED MICROSCOPY WITHIN A HOSPITAL

The POCT coordinator should be familiar with the locations at which PPM procedures are performed to be certain that appropriate CLIA licensure has been obtained for the physician responsible for these procedures. An alternative approach is to include PPM under the POCT program coordinated by the laboratory. Training of new residents could be undertaken on a day during their orientation. Kodachrome images may be used. The same slide file could be used to organize proficiency testing activity, or this goal may be achieved by purchasing the Excel program XL-G from the College of American Pathologists. Quality control materials are not available, as defined previously. Laboratories doing these tests are expected to follow good laboratory practices, however, in terms of quality control, quality assurance, and proficiency testing.

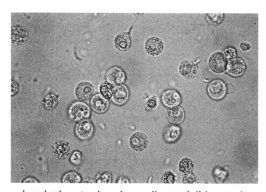

Fig. 5. Polymorphonuclear leukocytes in urine sediment (oil immersion, original magnification ×50).

Competency indicators for PPM might include monitoring the number of proficiency testing or blood sample testing failures or failed procedural observations.[37] The following list illustrates some of the perplexities encountered in the hospital-based application of PPM.

1. Specimen is labile; microscopy must be done without delay. Difficulties in reviewing findings by others.
2. No quality control materials are available. Quality control not part of quality-assurance program. Potential home-brew material to simulate fern test, for example.
3. Training of residents and existing staff.
4. Cost analysis—linked to outcomes.
5. Outcome analysis: Is length of stay decreased by PPM? What defect occurs if PPM is not performed or performed inadequately?
6. Data placed on chart manually or not all.

The connectivity solution for a POCT program would include a computer screen to record results so that they can be sent through an interface to the LIS/HIS.

The resolution of most of these issues depends on local policies, procedures, and politics.

ACKNOWLEDGMENTS

Thanks are extended to Pat Schmidt for typing the manuscript.

REFERENCES

1. Point-of-care testing, section 30. Northfield (IL): College of American Pathologists; 1997. p. 1–18.
2. Anonymous. The tests for albumen and sugar in the urine. [editorial]. Lancet 1893;i:956.
3. Arora VK, Singh N, Chaturvedi S, et al. Fine needle aspiration diagnosis of subcutaneous abscess from Enterobius vermicularis infestation. Acta Cytol 1997;41:1845–7.
4. Cushman WC. A century of indirect blood pressure measurement. Arch Intern Med 1996;156:1922–3.
5. Mar J, Pastor R, Abásolo R, et al. Ambulatory blood pressure monitoring and diagnostic errors in hypertension: a Bayesian approach. Med Decis Making 1998;18:429–35.
6. Shuler CL, Allison N, Holcomb S, et al. Accuracy of an automated blood pressure device in stable inpatients. Optimum versus routine use. Arch Intern Med 1998; 158:714–21.
7. Kiechle FL. Point-of-care testing. Washington, DC: American Association for Clinical Chemistry; 1998. p. 1–98.
8. Miller KA, Miller NA. Joining forces to improve point-of-care testing. Nurs Manag 1998;28:34–7.
9. Cembrowski GS, Kiechle FL. Point-of-care testing: critical analysis and practical application. Adv Pathol Lab Med 1994;7:3–26.
10. Ehrmeyer SS, Laessig RH. Regulatory requirements (CLIA '88, JCAHO, CAP) for decentralized testing. Am J Clin Pathol 1995;104(Suppl 1):S40–9.
11. Kiechle FL, Cembrowski G. Quality improvement in the critical care laboratory. Cht Care Rep 1991;2:282–94.
12. Kiechle FL, Ingram-Main R. Quality improvement and point-of-care testing. J Clin Ligand Assay 1995;18:14–20.

13. Methany NA, Clouse RE. Bedside methods for detecting aspiration in tube-fed patients. Chest 1997;111:724–31.
14. Methany NA, Smith L. pH, color and feeding tubes. RN 1998;61:25–7.
15. Provider-performed microscopy testing: proposed guideline. Wayne (PA): National Committee for Clinical Laboratory Standards HS2-P; 2000 h.
16. Ong YYT, Pintauro WM. Silver stools. JAMA 1979;242:2433.
17. Craig RM. Alimentary tract and excerine pancreas. In: Noe DA, Rock RC, editors. Laboratory medicine. The selection and interpretation of clinical laboratory studies. Baltimore (MD): Williams & Wilkins; 1994. p. 383–400.
18. Harrie JC, Dupont HL, Hornick RB. Fecal leukocytes in diarrhea illness. Ann Intern Med 1972;76:697–703.
19. Kao YS, Liu FJ-F, Alexander DR. Laboratory diagnosis of gastrointestinal tract and exocrine pancreatic disorders. In: Henry JB, editor. Clinical diagnosis and management by laboratory methods. Philadelphia: WB Saunders Co; 1996. p. 332–8.
20. Kjeldsberg CR, Knight JA. Amniotic fluid. In: Body fluids. Laboratory examination of amniotic, cerebrospinal, seminal, serous and synovial fluids. Chicago: American Society of Clinical Pathologists; 1993. p. 1–63.
21. Free AH, Free HM. Laboratory interrelationships of amniotic fluid and urine. In: Natelson S, Scommegna A, Epstein MB, editors. Amniotic fluid. New York: J Wiley & Sons; 1974. p. 37–46.
22. Addison A. Obstetrical ferning test. Lab Med 1999;30:451.
23. Gregg AR. Introduction to premature rupture of membranes. Obstet Gynecol Clin North Am 1992;19:241–9.
24. Peredy TR, Powers RD. Bedside diagnostic testing of body fluids. Am J Emerg Med 1997;15:400–7.
25. Smith RW, Callagen DA. Amniotic fluid crystallization test for ruptured membranes. Obstet Gynecol 1962;20:655–60.
26. Tietz N. Fundamentals of clinical chemistry. 3rd edition. Philadelphia: WB Saunders Co; 1987. p. 271–2.
27. Braat DD, Smeenk JM, Manger AP, et al. Saliva test as ovulation predictor. Lancet 1998;352:1283–4.
28. Ringsrud KM, Linné JJ. Body fluids. In: Urinalysis and body fluids. A color text and atlas. St. Louis (MO): Mobsy-Year Books, Inc; 1995. p. 206–13.
29. Sinton E. Seminal fluid. In: Kjeldsberg CR, Knight JA, editors. Body fluids. Laboratory examination of amniotic, cerebrospinal, seminal, serous and synovial fluids. Chicago: American Society of Clinical Pathologists; 1993. p. 255–64.
30. Jones HW Jr, Toner JP. The infertile couple. N Engl J Med 1993;329:1710–5.
31. Collins KA. The laboratory's role in detecting sexual assault. Lab Med 1998;29:361–5.
32. Baker DJ, Paterson MA, Klaassen JM, et al. Semen evaluations in the clinical laboratory. How well are they being performed? Lab Med 1994;25:509–14.
33. Beattie RM, Walker-Smith JA, Domizio P. Ileal and colonic ulceration due to enterobiasis. J Pediatr Gastroenterol Nutr 1995;21:232–4.
34. Adelman MM. Sperm morphology. Lab Med 1986;17:32–4.
35. Davis RO, Baen DE, Siemers RJ, et al. Accuracy and precision of the CellForm-Human automated sperm morphometry instrument. Fertil Steril 1992;58:763–9.
36. Mahmoud AM, Depoorter B, Piens N, et al. The performance of 10 different methods for the estimation of sperm concentration. Fertil Steril 1997;68:340–5.
37. Gerrity M. Guidelines for human andrology laboratories. Fertil Steril 1992;58(Suppl 1):11S–6S.

38. Pool TB. Practices contributing to quality performance in the embryo laboratory and the status of laboratory regulation in the US. Hum Reprod 1997;12:2591–3.
39. Van Riper G. Pyrantel pamoate for pinworm infestation. Am Pharm 1993;NS33: 43–4.
40. Ok UZ, Ertan P, Limoncu E, et al. Relationship between pinworm and urinary tract infections in young girls. APMIS 1999;107:474–6.
41. Mishriki Y. Dealing with the unexpected nematode. Postgrad Med 1997;102:37–8.
42. Avolio L, Avoltini V, Ceffa F, et al. Perianal granuloma caused by *Enterobius vermicularis*: report of a new observation and review of the literature. J Pediatr 1998; 132:1055–6.
43. Schmidt G, Roberts L. Foundations of parasitology. 4th edition. St. Louis (MO): Times Mirror/Mosby College Publishing; 1989. p. 464–9.
44. Schumann GGB, Schweitzer SC. Examination of urine. In: Henry JB, editor. Clinical and diagnosis management by laboratory methods. 18th edition. Philadelphia: WB Saunders Co; 1991. p. 387–444.
45. Maslamani S, Glenton PA, Khan SR. Changes in urine macromolecular composition during processing. J Urol 2000;164:230–6.
46. Millar L, Debuque L, Leialoha AG, et al. Rapid enzymatic urine screening test to detect bacteriuria in pregnancy. Obstet Gynecol 2000;95:601–4.
47. Joint Commission. Quality point of care testing. A joint commission handbook. Oakbrook Terrace (IL): JCAHO; 1999. p. 41–73.

Point-of-Care Testing for Disasters: Needs Assessment, Strategic Planning, and Future Design

Gerald J. Kost, MD, PhD, MS, FACB*, Kristin N. Hale, BS, BA,
T. Keith Brock, BS, Richard F. Louie, PhD, Nicole L. Gentile, BS,
Tyler K. Kitano, BS, Nam K. Tran, PhD

- Biohazard containment • Hurricane Katrina
- Modular test design • Newdemics • Sampling method
- Small-world network (SWN) • Tsunami

GOALS AND OBJECTIVES

The goals of point-of-care testing (POCT) are to facilitate rapid evidence-based decisions, to improve patient outcomes, and, ultimately, to be robust and reliable enough for on-site applications in emergency and disaster settings worldwide.

The objectives of this article are (1) to review current POC technologies used in disaster and emergency care, (2) to understand first responder needs, (3) to outline device design criteria based on gap analysis, and (4) to present strategies for improving future POCT for efficiency, effectiveness, and targeted treatment during on-site field operations.

This article is evidence-based in that it presents preliminary results of a needs assessment survey in the United States. Readers are encouraged to participate in the needs assessment survey. Please see the instructions provided in **Table 1**.

This study was supported by the Point-of-Care Testing Center for Teaching and Research (POCT•CTR^SM), School of Medicine, University of California, Davis, and by a NIBIB Point-of-Care Technologies Center grant (Dr Kost, PI, NIH U54 EB007959). The content is solely the responsibility of the authors and does not necessarily represent the official views of the National Institute of Biomedical Imaging and Bioengineering or the National Institutes of Health.
Department of Pathology and Laboratory Medicine, UC Davis-LLNL Point-of-Care Technologies Center [NIBIB, NIH], Point-of-Care Testing Center for Teaching and Research (POCT•CTR), School of Medicine, University of California, 3455 Tupper Hall, Davis, CA 95616, USA
* Corresponding author.
E-mail address: gjkost@ucdavis.edu (G.J. Kost).

Clin Lab Med 29 (2009) 583–605
doi:10.1016/j.cll.2009.07.014
labmed.theclinics.com
0272-2712/09/$ – see front matter © 2009 Elsevier Inc. All rights reserved.

Table 1
SurveyMonkey Instructions

Step	Instruction and Access
One	Visit UC Davis-LLNL POCT. Web site: http://www.ucdmc.ucdavis.edu/pathology/poctcenter
Two	The Clinical Needs Assessment survey link appears in the top right corner of the navigation bar. It is the first item under POC Technologies Center. Please click on "Needs Assessment Survey"
Three	Please contact Keith Brock, Research Specialist, at 530 752 8471, email: tkbrock@ucdavis.edu, to receive an accession number
Four	Follow the instructions on the screen to complete the survey. *Note:* Your progress will be saved after pressing the "next" button at the end of each page. Please note, your progress online is managed through your web browser cookies. Please complete the survey on the same computer and do not delete the cookies on your web browser before completion of the online survey
Five	Thank you for your time and input on the survey!

The 2004 tsunami in Southeast Asia and Hurricane Katrina in the United States exposed the lack of disaster preparedness worldwide.[1] Although the feasibility of POCT was proven, and the disaster responses were extensive, follow-up studies showed rescue was slow and inadequate.[1] In Hurricane Katrina, flooded hospitals, roads, and communications hindered rescue efforts by first responders who carried limited POCT devices such as oxygen saturation monitors (pulse oximeters), blood glucose meters, and other small handhelds.[1] Furthermore, POCT instruments failed to operate effectively under adverse environmental conditions at respective disaster locations, where temperatures reached 110°F (43°C) or higher in hospitals.[2,3]

Broadly regional catastrophes, such as these recent "newdemics,"[4,5] lead to sequentially magnified setbacks. Others, such as the current novel H1N1 pandemic, threaten entire nations. Typically, communities lack the POCT resources necessary to effectively handle the disaster situations they face.[1] Conversely, newdemics highlight the significant potential for POCT to positively impact preparedness, disaster response, and patient outcomes. Current experiences, including the surprise appearance of the novel H1N1 pandemic in Mexico (unpublished observation), emphasize the need for new sturdy, handheld, and robust POC technologies capable of effectively operating in a variety of field locations.

In the future, better prepared first responders will carry reliable POCT diagnostics wherever disaster and emergency situations arise. Thus, POC user needs are being established through objective evidence-based national surveys (see **Table 1**) as a first step in identifying suitable device designs, effective test clusters, and environmental operating conditions.[6] The preliminary survey results are reported.

NEEDS ASSESSMENT SURVEY: PRELIMINARY RESULTS
Participants

Forty disaster care experts were randomly selected from the editorial boards of the *American Journal of Disaster Medicine* (AJDM) and *Disaster Medicine Public Health and Preparedness* (DMPHP) using a random number generator (Minitab, State College, PA). This sample included physicians, public health officials, researchers, pathologists, first responders, and military personnel.

Development

A survey was developed based on literature review and multidisciplinary consultations that included professors of bioengineering, emergency medicine, infectious diseases, and critical care medicine. "Visual logistics," defined as graphics and pictorial media for common sense portrayal of questions, concepts, and designs, are introduced to build survey questions with the objective of generating easy to comprehend concepts without laborious text or lengthy explanation. Set theory (eg, Venn diagrams) was used whenever possible to compare 2 or more visual concepts, questions, and the results.

To encourage participation and simplify distribution and return, a visual logistics web-based survey was developed (SurveyMonkey, Portland, Oregon). Paper-based and web-based surveys used identical graphics and questions. The survey was divided into 4 parts: (1) demographic questions, (2) device design questions in 10 sections, (3) pathogen test cluster design questions in 4 sections, and (4) trade-off blocks that led to heuristic ranking of POC design features. At the time of this preliminary report, parts 1 to 3 were implemented.

Procedures

If possible, personal contact was initiated by phone followed by shipment of a FedEx package containing an invitation letter, the paper-based survey, and a prepaid return envelope. The invitation letter explained the goal of the survey, provided instructions for participation, and included a hyperlink to the web-based survey (see **Table 1**). Email also was used to distribute the survey request and hyperlink. This preliminary report reflects survey results obtained between March 1 and June 14, 2009. The survey was conducted in compliance with the UC Davis Institutional Review Board.

Statistics

Data obtained from the survey were analyzed using nonparametric Pearson chi-square exact tests (SAS, Gary, North Carolina). Statistical significance was defined as: $*$, $P<.05$; $**$, $P<.01$; and $***$, $P<.001$.

Pathogen test cluster rank results were analyzed by assigning each pathogen a weighted score. The score for each rank was calculated using the following equation: $S_i = (11 - R_i)$. R_i is defined as the rank of each pathogen assigned by a survey participant, such that $i = [1, n]$, where n is the number of ranks. When the respondent designated the same rank for 2 or more organisms, the average rank was calculated and assigned to each organism.

The weighted score was calculated by summing the product of each score and corresponding frequency using the following equation: $WS_j = \sum_{i=1} S_i \times F_{ij}$. The frequency, F_{ij} is defined as the number of times survey participants ranked a pathogen a specific value, such that $j = [1, N]$, where N is the number of pathogens.

PRELIMINARY RESULTS

Demography

Of the 40 disaster medicine experts surveyed, 25 responses were received, giving a response rate of 62%. The respondents included 8 physicians (32%), 9 public health officials/hospital managers (36%), 3 pathologists (12%), and 5 emergency room doctors (20%).

Device Design

Fig. 1 illustrates visual logistics, specifically pictorial media that introduced the survey question on what the respondent preferred with regard to instrument formats for

TRANSPORTABLE   PORTABLE   HANDHELD

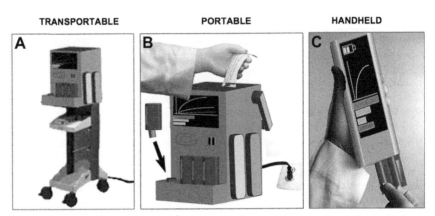

Fig. 1. Device design format. Visual logistics were used to illustrate 3 device format selections for POCT instruments. (*A*) Transportable device on a cart. (*B*) Portable, bench-top device with a handle for carrying. (*C*) Small battery-operated handheld device.

given clinical settings. The results showed that in disaster settings, respondents showed a significant preference for handheld diagnostics (**Fig. 2**) and cited increased portability and versatility as the rationale.

When respondents were asked to choose between a device that tests multiple patient samples in parallel for a single pathogen versus a device that performs multiplex testing of several pathogens for a single patient sample (**Fig. 3**), respondents preferred a multiplex test in the urgent care and emergency room settings (**Fig. 4**). Participants cited the need to quickly screen a large volume of patients in a disaster setting, whereas a full workup is necessary in urgent care and emergency room settings. Several of the respondents who chose the device that parallel processes

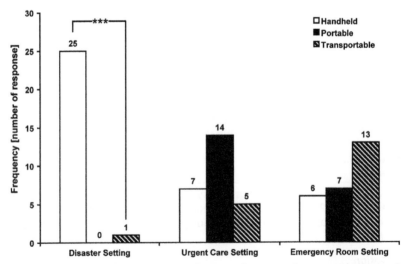

Fig. 2. Selection of format by survey respondents. In disaster settings, participants preferred handheld devices (***$P<.001$). For urgent care and emergency-room settings, there were no statistically significant differences in preferences.

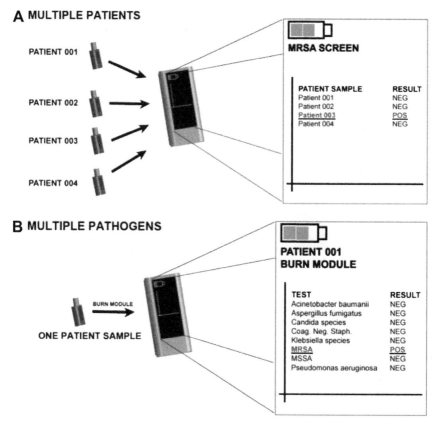

Fig. 3. Multiple patients versus multiplex pathogens. Visual logistics were used to illustrate 2 testing methods for POCT devices. (*A*) Testing multiple patients for 1 pathogen. (*B*) Multiplex pathogen testing, in which 1 patient sample is simultaneously tested for the presence of multiple pathogens (*underline*).

multiple patient samples for a single pathogen given a disaster setting, referenced biothreat or pandemic scenarios.

Fig. 5 shows 2 different sample collection methods, a test cassette and vacutainer. A test cassette provides a housing platform in which one can automate preanalytical processing steps that are critical to subsequent analytical steps that follow on the POC device. **Fig. 6** reflects general acceptance of test cassettes in disaster, urgent care, and emergency settings.

Respondents were also asked to state their preference between 2 potential waste disposal methods (**Fig. 7**). The first scheme suggests an instrument that stores biohazard waste in a reusable waste storage reservoir to be emptied periodically. A test cassette, used to transport the sample to the instrument, would also need to be properly discarded after a single use. The second scheme shows an instrument that stores all biohazard waste in the disposable test cassette, which then is discarded after a single use. **Fig. 8** shows a statistically significant preference of respondents for the disposable test cassette in the second scheme across all 3 clinical settings, with a higher level of statistical significance ($P<.01$) of the preference in disaster and emergency room settings.

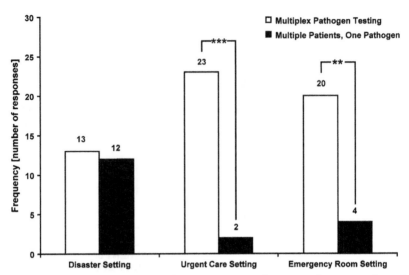

Fig. 4. Selection of testing method by survey respondents. In disaster settings, both approaches to pathogen detection may be useful. However, respondents preferred multiplex testing to testing multiple patients for 1 pathogen in urgent care (***P<.001) and emergency room (**P<.01) settings.

Pathogen Test Cluster Design

Table 2 shows the weighted scores of the top 10 pathogens for each of 4 scenario sections. For a general disaster test cluster, *Vibrio cholerae* had the highest weighted score (117); whereas for a blood donor screening test cluster, HIV 1 and 2 had the highest weighted score (224). Depending on the clinical scenario, the specific

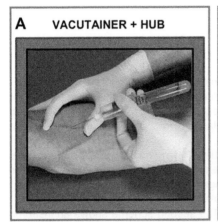
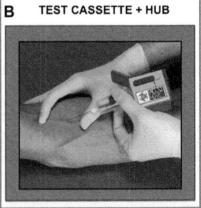

Fig. 5. Test cassettes versus vacutainers. Visual logistics were used to illustrate 2 sample collection methods for POCT instruments. (*A*) A vacutainer is used to collect the blood sample, allowing for multiple blood collection tubes to be drawn at one time. (*B*) Test cassette blood sample collection; blood is drawn directly into a disposable test cassette, processed, and a result given. Graphics updated for the survey currently in use.

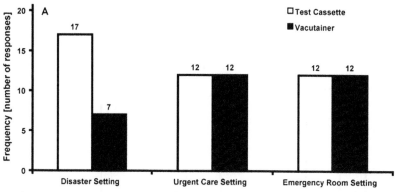

Fig. 6. Selection of sample collection method by survey respondents. Test cassettes and vacutainers were equivalent in all but the disaster setting, but this result was not statistically significant in this preliminary survey report.

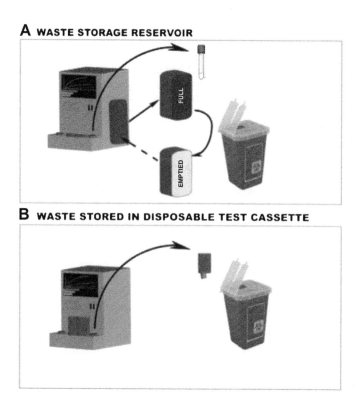

Fig. 7. Biohazard disposal methods. Visual logistics were used to illustrate 2 biohazard disposal methods for POCT devices. (*A*) Biohazard waste in a reusable waste storage reservoir that must be emptied periodically, and a disposable test cassette for single use. (*B*) A device that stores all biohazard waste in a disposable test cassette that is discarded after a single use. Graphics updated for the survey currently in use.

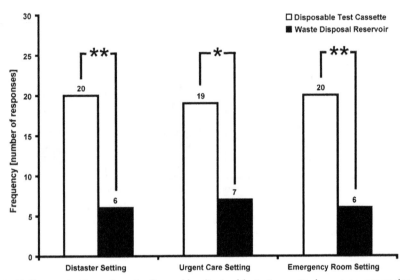

Fig. 8. Uniform selection of waste disposal by disposable test cassette by survey respondents. There is a statistically significant preference for disposable test cassettes across all 3 clinical settings (P<.01, 0.05, and 0.01). See **Fig. 6**. Disposable test cassettes have merit for sample collection and waste disposal in disaster settings. *P<.05; **P<.01.

pathogens a POC device would detect varies. For instance, methicillin-resistant *Staphylococcus aureus* (MRSA) had the highest weighted score at 147 for the bloodstream pathogen test cluster (see **Table 2**). However, in the pandemic test cluster, influenza A/B had the highest weighted score at 189, whereas MRSA was fifth with a weighted score of 112.5 (see **Table 2**).

PRELIMINARY RESULTS VERSUS CURRENT DISASTER PATHOGENS

Various POCT devices that test for a variety of analytes and pathogens are used during disaster and emergency situations, such as Hurricane Katrina. Emergency medical responders, disaster medical assistance teams (DMATs), international medical-surgical response teams (IMSuRTs), and other first responders deploy to disaster sites carrying POCT devices.[6] They use POCT devices to test, rapidly diagnose, and, as indicated, treat victims.[6] Depending on where responders are deployed, the pathogens they encounter will vary, possibly unpredictably and unexpectedly. **Table 3**[7–32] documents the variety of pathogens present in several modern disasters, such as flooding, hurricanes, and earthquakes. When comparing the top 10 pathogens identified by preliminary needs assessment survey results in various disaster scenarios (see **Table 2**) with pathogens found in major disasters, there was substantial overlap.

During Hurricane Katrina, for example, various pathogens were identified that also were selected and ranked by experts and surveyed as high priority for general disaster, blood donor screening, bloodstream pathogen, and pandemic test clusters. Specifically, in **Table 2** for the general disaster scenario and in **Table 3** for Hurricane Katrina, there is overlap for *Vibrio cholerae*, MRSA, and *Escherichia coli*. Thus, preliminary survey results demonstrate that survey experts identified pathogens encountered at disaster sites (see **Table 3**) as important for having POCT devices capable of detecting these organisms (see **Table 2**).

Table 2
Pathogen test clusters

	Weighted Score	Pathogen
A. General disaster	117	*Vibrio cholerae*
test cluster (n = 18)	108	*Escherichia coli*
	100	*Staphylococcus aureus*
	77	Yellow fever
	73	*Salmonella enterica*
	66	*Pseudomonas aeruginosa*
	62	*Plasmodium falciparum*
	54	*Enterobacter* species
	49	Dengue fever virus
	38	*Klebsiella* species
B. Blood donor screening	224	HIV 1 and 2
test cluster (n = 23)	190	Hepatitis B
	190	Hepatitis C
	125.5	Human T cell lymphotropic virus 1 and 2 (HTLV 1 and 2)
	109.5	West Nile virus
	109	*Cytomegalovirus*
	93	Dengue fever
	77	Parvovirus B19
	74	Epstein-Barr virus
	46	Chikungunya
C. Bloodstream pathogen	147	Methicillin-resistant *Staphylococcus aureus*
test cluster (n = 20)	118	*Escherichia coli*
	91	*Pseudomonas aeruginosa*
	90.5	*Streptococcus pneumoniae*
	90	*Enterobacter* species
	87.5	Methicillin-sensitive *Staphylococcus aureus*
	79	*Klebsiella* species
	61	*Enterococcus faecalis*
	50	*Streptococcus pyogenes*
	48	Coagulase-negative *Staphylococcus*
D. Pandemic test	189	*Influenza A/B*
cluster (n = 22)	121.5	*Parainfluenza 1, 2, 3*
	115.5	*Streptococcus pneumoniae*
	112.5	Respiratory syncytial virus
	112.5	Methicillin-resistant *Staphylococcus aureus*
	100	*Haemophilus influenza*
	90.5	*Mycobacterium tuberculosis*
	87	Adenovirus
	57	*Mycoplasm pneumoniae*
	51.5	Metapneumovirus

A similar finding was observed when comparing pathogens detected at the tsunami disaster site in Southeast Asia (see **Table 3**) versus the general disaster and bloodstream pathogen test clusters ranked highly in **Table 2**. Survey results identified several pathogens in the general disaster and bloodstream pathogen test clusters, such as *Escherichia coli*, *Klebsiella pneumoniae*, *Pseudomonas aeruginosa*, MRSA, and *Salmonella* species. These pathogens also were detected at tsunami disaster sites in Southeast Asia. Having POCT devices capable of testing for these pathogens found at particular disaster sites can facilitate rapid diagnosis. Targeted therapy, in turn, can conserve drugs (eg, antimicrobials) that become depleted quickly during the initial crisis stages. These survey results should be used as a guide for development of new POCT devices capable of timely pathogen detection at disaster sites.

CURRENT USE OF POCT IN DISASTERS IN THE UNITED STATES

New POC devices must be capable of testing for a variety of pathogens present at a particular disaster site, and also properly integrated and used to decrease response

Table 3
Pathogens in disasters

Scenario	Location, Year	Pathogens Detected (Isolation Site)	Path of Infection
Drought	Florida, 5 epidemics since 1952[7,8]	Saint Louis encephalitis (blood)	Vector borne
		West Nile (blood)	Vector borne
	Indonesia, 1997[9]	Malaria (blood)	Vector borne
Earthquake	California, 1994[10]	*Coccidioides immitis* (skin)	Dust cloud
	China, 2008[11]	*Staphylococcus aureus* (pus and wound)	Wound
		Escherichia coli (pus and wound)	Wound
		Acinetobacter baumannii (pus and wound)	Wound
		Enterobacter cloacae (pus and wound)	Wound
		Pseudomonas aeruginosa (pus and wound)	Wound
	Turkey, 1999[12]	*Pseudomonas aeruginosa* (wound)	Wound
		Acinetobacter baumannii (wound)	Wound
		Methicillin-resistant *Staphylococcus aureus* (wound)	Wound
		Candida species (wound)	Wound
	Turkey, 1999[13]	*Acinetobacter* species (wound)	Wound
		Pseudomonas aeruginosa (wound, blood, urine)	Wound
		Methicillin-resistant *Staphylococcus aureus* (wound, blood, urine)	Wound
		Serratia marcescens (wound)	Wound
		Klebsiella pneumoniae (wound)	Wound
		Enterobacter species (wound)	Wound
		Candida albicans (wound)	Wound
Flooding	Bangladesh, 2004[14]	*Escherichia coli* (blood)	Water, food borne
		Vibrio cholerae (stool)	
	Global, 1980–2008[15]	Malaria (blood)	Vector borne
		Yellow fever (blood)	Vector borne
		West Nile (blood)	Vector borne
		Dengue (blood)	Vector borne
	Indonesia, 2004[16]	*Salmonella paratyphi* (blood)	Water, food borne
	Nonspecific[17,18]	*Streptococcus pneumoniae* (blood)	Inhalation

(continued on next page)

Table 3
(continued)

Scenario	Location, Year	Pathogens Detected (Isolation Site)	Path of Infection
Hurricanes/ tornadoes	Katrina, 2005[19–23]	Nontoxigenic *Vibrio cholerae* O1 (blood)	Food borne
		Vibrio cholerae non-O1 (blood)	Water borne
		Vibrio vulnificus (blood)	Wound, food borne
		Vibrio parahaemolyticus (blood)	Wound, food borne
		Methicillin-resistant *Staphylococcus aureus* (wound)	Wound
		Norovirus (stool)	Water borne
		Vibrio species (lake surface water)	Water borne
		Legionella species (lake surface water)	Water borne
		Cryptosporidium (interior canal water)	Water borne
		Giardia (interior canal water)	Water borne
		Escherichia coli (shoreline canal water)	Water borne
		Bifidobacterium (shoreline canal water)	Water borne
	Georgia, 2000[24]	*Serratia marcescens* (wound)	Wound
		Pseudomonas aeruginosa (wound)	Wound
		Enterococcus (wound)	Wound
Low-resource settings/ rural areas	Indonesia, 2001–2003[16]	*Salmonella enterica* (blood)	Food, water borne
		Salmonella paratyphi (blood)	Food, water borne
		Salmonella typhi (blood)	Food, water borne
	Philippines, 1994–1996[25]	*Streptococcus pneumoniae* (blood)	Inhalation
		Haemophilus influenzae (blood)	Inhalation
Tsunamis	Thailand, 2004[26–29]	*Aeromonas* (pus and wound)	Wound
		Escherichia coli (stool)	Water, food borne
		Klebsiella pneumoniae (pus and wound)	Wound
		Pseudomonas aeruginosa (pus and wound)	Wound
		Burkolderia pseudomallei (blood)	Soil, water borne
		Acinetobacter baumannii (blood)	Soil, water borne
		Stenotrophomonas (blood)	Soil, water borne
		Methicillin-resistant *Staphylococcus aureus* (wound)	Wound
		Staphylococcus aureus (wound)	Wound
		Candida species (blood)	Inhalation, wound
		Aspergillus species (blood)	Inhalation, wound
		Scedosporium species (blood)	Inhalation, wound
		Salmonella species (well water)	Water borne
		Clostridium species (wound)	Soil
		Aeromonas species (wound)	Water borne
World Trade Center disaster	New York, 2001[30–32]	Asthma and WTC cough (pathogens not named)	

US Army 14th Combat Support Hospital

US Navy

Ortho-Diagnostics Blood Typing: ABO Blood Group

Cardiac STATus: cTnI, CK-MB, Myoglobin

US Army 14th Combat Support Hospital

US Military, Local Surveyed Hospital

Rapidpoint Coag: PT, aPTT, Heparin Management Test

i-STAT: ACT, PT/INR, glucose, creatinine, cTnI, Na^+, K^+, Cl^-, Ca^{++}, pH, pCO_2, pO_2, SO_2, Hct, Hb, BUN, CK-MB, BNP

Hospitals, Evacuation Sites

US Army, Navy, Marine Corps

Piccolo: Albumin, ALP, ALT, amylase, AST, BUN, creatinine, Ca, Cl , K , Na , Mg, LD, HDL, cholesterol, triglycerides, CK, glucose, TP, phosphorous, total bilirubin, direct bilirubin, TCO_2, GGT, uric acid

Capillary Blood Glucose Meters

US Air Force

Triage

Cardiac Panel: cTnI, CK-MB, myoglobin

Drugs of Abuse: Amphetamines, Methamphetamines

Donation to Local Red Cross

45,000 Blood Glucose Meters

e patient outcomes. During Hurricane Katrina, a variety of different
es of POCT were used featuring an array of POC tests covering
ology, and other analyte categories.

POC instruments, including the various locations and POCT oper-
Katrina. Hospitals, evacuation sites, and local agencies were not
disaster and offered few POCT devices and tests. Hurricane Katrina
a newdemic.[5] Supplies depleted quickly. Needs for chronic moni-
atpatient glucose monitoring, were not met.

Hurricane Katrina disaster sites, arrival, and responses of mostly
nd a suggested optimal POCT plan (upper right in figure) for timely
e. **Fig. 10** also documents that the disaster response time was
CT disaster preparation does not meet adequate standards and
d for future preparedness. Proper strategic placement of POCT,
ate medical care facilities, is needed to facilitate rapid diagnosis

enza strains, such as novel H1N1, have the potential to significantly
and morbidity, as well as quickly deplete resources of current health
es. Thus, for example, rapidly diagnosing a particular influenza strain
ces is advantageous. Furthermore, the World Health Organization
recommends the use of POCT devices for quick influenza
nercially available POC tests for influenza A and B are listed in
eral of the tests currently available are immunoassays that target
natrix protein to identify influenza A or B types, but rarely offer further

ic acid recognition (NAR) for detection of influenza A or B has shown
s (see **Table 4**). These NAR devices exhibit greater sensitivity and
ping data. Once a subtype of influenza is positively identified, health
d public health workers have the ability to start surveillance of new
ular area. In addition, subtyping of influenza has the ability to guide
t by identifying particular influenza strains that may be resistant or
al treatment.

---

d types of POCT in Hurricane Katrina. Hospitals, evacuation sites, and local
prepared fully to assist quickly with POCT. They carried few POCT instru-
US military ships and combat support units were equipped with POCT
a variety of tests to facilitate rapid diagnosis and treatment. Donations
roved valuable, but not fast enough or adequate for the large numbers
involved in the disaster. POC tests used during the disaster include: ALP,
se; ALT, alanine aminotransferase; aPTT, activated partial thromboplastin
e aminotransferase; BNP, B-type natriuretic peptide; BUN, blood (serum)
creatine kinase; cTn, cardiac troponin; GGT, γ-glutamyltransferase; Hb,
ematocrit; HDL, high-density lipoprotein; INR, international normalized
hydrogenase; MB, MB fraction of CK; PT, prothrombin time; SO$_2$, oxygen
d by pulse oximetry; TCO$_2$, total carbon dioxide content; TP, total protein.
ications: Bayer Acsensia, http://www.bayercarediabetes.com; Cardiac
v.spectraldx.com; Cell-Dyn, http://www.abbottdiagnostics.com; i-STAT,
om; Ortho Diagnostics blood typing, http://www.orthoclinical.com;
.abaxis.com; Rapidpoint coag, http://www.bayer-poct.co.uk; and Triage,

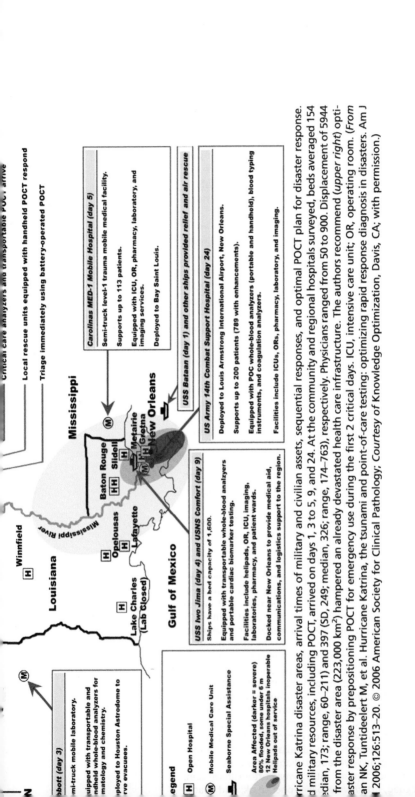

...rricane Katrina disaster areas, arrival times of military and civilian assets, sequential responses, and optimal POCT plan for disaster response. ...d military resources, including POCT, arrived on days 1, 3 to 5, 9, and 24. At the community and regional hospitals surveyed, beds averaged 154 ...edian, 173; range, 60–211) and 397 (SD, 249; median, 326; range, 174–763), respectively. Physicians ranged from 50 to 900. Displacement of 5944 ...from the disaster area (223,000 km²) hampered an already devastated health care infrastructure. The authors recommend (*upper right*) opti-...aster response by prepositioning POCT for emergency use during the first 2 critical days. ICU, intensive care unit; OR, operating room. (*From* ...an NK, Tuntideelert M, et al. Hurricane Katrina, the tsunami and point-of-care testing: optimizing rapid response diagnosis in disasters. Am J ...2006;126:513–20. © 2006 American Society for Clinical Pathology; *Courtesy of Knowledge Optimization, Davis, CA;* with permission.)

For instance, several H1N1 strains of influenza were resistant to oseltamivir in fall 2008; however, in spring 2009, the novel H1N1 influenza strain ("swine flu") was sensitive to oseltamivir. Furthermore, in a recent study conducted by Dr Nishiura and colleagues,[39] the use of quarantine and rapid diagnostic testing to prevent or delay the spread of pandemic influenza across island nations was evaluated. In order for quarantine strategy to be effective in preventing or delaying the spread of pandemic influenza, rapid and reliable diagnostic testing must be used to positively identify index cases (first victims) with influenza.[39] Thus, the use of POCT to rapidly diagnose and subtype influenza has significant potential to refine pandemic disaster response and prevent newdemics from spreading outside the bounds of initial disaster or emergency locations.

This concept is important for disasters on the horizon, such as extensively drug-resistant malaria and tuberculosis. Globally, tuberculosis represents a major problem, especially in low-resource settings, such as impoverished African nations. Current tests available often fail to correctly identify tuberculosis, are not rapid, and cannot identify drug resistance.[40] Rapid-liquid culture shows promising results for tuberculosis detection by improving the sensitivity, speed, reliability, and multidrug-resistant tuberculosis detection.[40] Future thinking is required for developing POCT devices that are proven to simultaneously be rapid, simple, reliable, and cost-effective for diagnosing extensively drug-resistant tuberculosis.[40]

PREPAREDNESS: GAP ANALYSIS

POCT devices typically encounter harsh environmental conditions, temperature extremes, and high humidity in emergency and disaster care. Despite substantial improvements, gaps still exist between current POCT technologies and real-world needs. Inability of POCT instruments and reagents to withstand harsh conditions present at disaster and emergency sites compromises performance.[6] For example, glucose test strips and blood gas cartridges may not provide accurate measurements at disaster sites because thermal stresses adversely and inconsistently affect performance.[6] Because of these types of limitations and the obvious technical gaps in POC devices as we know them today, the United States and other countries are not prepared for disasters.

Box 1 highlights gaps between current POC devices and various problems with technologies currently available. Without durable and robust POCT equipment, diagnosis and treatment of victims at disaster sites becomes increasingly complicated and hindered. To effectively and efficiently diagnose, monitor, and treat patients, the current gaps in POCT technologies and devices must be closed. The POC Technologies Center (http://www.ucdmc.ucdavis.edu/pathology/poctcenter) is currently conducting static and dynamic environmental stress tests to understand the environmental limitations of POC devices and reagents in more detail.

Dynamic tests simulate realistic meteorologic conditions found in world regions with high risk for newdemics. US Food and Drug Administration (FDA)-approved product labelings typically state temperature limits, but current limits are inadequate for most disaster conditions. Also, a POCT method that may be proven to work in environmental extremes must also be validated for critically ill patient populations, which few currently do.

Problems with preanalytical processing present an additional major challenge for reliable POCT device performance. For example, in a recent study conducted by Dighe and colleagues,[41] unusually high false-positive potassium critical values led the laboratory to investigate the preanalytical processing after concluding that the

Table 4
POC influenza diagnostic tests

Instrument/Manufacturer Immunoassay Tests	Type	Target	Time	Performance Characteristics (%)			
				Sensitivity	Specificity	PPV	NPV
3M Rapid Detection Flu A+B[34,a] http://www.3M.com, St. Paul, MN	Chromatographic immunoassay	Influenza A / Influenza B (nucleoprotein)	15 min	70 / 87	100 / 99	99 / 88	93 / 98
BD Directigen EZ Flu A+B,[a,b] http://www.bd.com, Franklin Lakes, NJ	Chromatographic immunoassay	Influenza A / Influenza B	15 min	77–91 / 69–100	86–99 / 99–100	60–98 / 93–98	93–95 / 93–100
BD Directigen Flu A Kit[a,b] http://www.bd.com, Franklin Lakes, NJ	Immunoassay	Influenza A (nucleoprotein)	15 min	67–96	88–97	NA	NA
BD Directigen Flu A + BKit[35,b] http://www.bd.com, Franklin Lakes, NJ	Immunoassay	Influenza A / Influenza B (nucleoprotein)	15 min	77–96 / 71–88	90–91 / 98–100	63–71 / 82–100	94–99 / 98–100
BinaxNOW Influenza A&B[36,a,b,c] http://www.binax.com, Scarborough, ME	Chromatographic immunoassay	Influenza A / Influenza B (nucleoprotein)	15 min	77–83 / 50–69	96–99 / 100	88–97 / 82–100	95–96 / 99
ESPLINE Influenza A&B,[36] http://www.fujirebio.co.jp, Tokyo, Japan	Chromatographic immunoassay	Influenza A / Influenza B (nucleoprotein)	15 min	67 / 30	100 / 100	100 / 100	89 / 96
fluID Rapid Influenza Test,[d] http://www.hxdiagnostics.com, Emeryville, CA	Lateral flow immunoassay	Influenza A / Influenza B / Subtype A/H1 / Subtype A/H3	NA / NA / NA / NA	NA / NA / NA / NA	NA / NA / NA / NA	NA / NA / NA / NA	NA / NA / NA / NA
Influ-A&B Respi-Strip, http://www.corisbio.com, Gembloux, Belgium	Chromatographic immunoassay	Influenza A / Influenza B (nucleoprotein)	15 min	97 / 97	100 / 100	100 / 100	98 / 98

Product	Method	Target	Time				
OSOM Influenza A & B Test,[a,c] http://www.genzymediagnostics.com, Framingham, MA	Chromatographic immunoassay	Influenza A	10 min	74	96	90	90
		Influenza B (nucleoprotein)		60	96	73	94
panfluID Rapid Influenza Test,[d] http://www.hxdiagnostics.com, Emeryville, CA	Lateral flow immunoassay	Avian Influenza	NA	NA	NA	NA	NA
QuickVue Influenza A+B Test,[c] http://www.quidel.com, San Diego, CA	Lateral flow immunoassay	Influenza A	10 min	77–94	89–99	62–91	95–99
		Influenza B (nucleoprotein)		62–82	97–99	80–90	94–97
QuickVue Influenza Test,[b,c] http://www.quidel.com, San Diego, CA	Lateral flow immunoassay	Influenza A+B No differentiation (nucleoprotein)	10 min	73–81	96–99	92–96	85–93
Rockeby Influenza A Test,[36,b] http://www.rockeby.com, Singapore	Immunoassay	Influenza A (nucleoprotein)	10 min	10	100	100	74
SAS FluAlert, http://www.sascientific.com, San Antonio, TX	Chromatographic immunoassay	Influenza A	15 min	76	98	93	91
		Influenza B (nucleoprotein)	15 min	91	99–100	100	99
Xpect Flu A&B Test Kit,[37] http://www.remelinc.com, Lenexa, KS	Chromatographic immunoassay	Influenza A	15 min	90–100	100	100	97–100
		Influenza B (nucleoprotein)		83–100	100	100	99–100
Nucleic Acid Tests							
Primer design, http://www.primerdesign.co.uk, Southampton, UK	Real time qPCR	H1N1 (swine flu)	<2 h	NA	NA	NA	NA
proFLU plus,[b] http://www.prodesse.com, Waukesha, WI	Real time RT-PCR	Influenza A (matrix)	3 h	100	93	71	100
		Influenza B (nonstructural NS1 & NS2)		98	99	80	100

(continued on next page)

Table 4
(continued)

| Instrument/Manufacturer | | | | Performance Characteristics (%) | | | |
Nucleic Acid Tests	Type	Target	Time	Sensitivity	Specificity	PPV	NPV
xTAG Respiratory viral panel,[38,a] Luminex, http://www.luminexcorp.com, Austin, TX	Flow through microsphere array	Influenza A	<4 h	98	100	99	100
		H1					
		H3					
		H5[b]					
		Influenza B		94	100	100	100
		SARS[b]					
		Corona virus NL63[b]					
		Corona virus 229E[b]					
		Corona virus OC43[b]					
		Corona virus HKU1[b]					
		RSV, subtype A					
		RSV, subtype B					
		Parainfluenza 1					
		Parainfluenza 2					
		Parainfluenza 3					
		Parainfluenza 4[b]					
		Metapneumovirus					
		Rhinovirus/					
		Enterovirus					
		Adenovirus					

Data shown in the table are from product inserts unless otherwise noted.

Abbreviations: BD, Becton-Dickinson; NA, not available; NPV, negative predictive value; PPV, positive predictive value; qPCR, quantitative polymerase chain reaction; RSV, respiratory syncytial virus; RT, reverse transcriptase; SARS, severe acute respiratory syndrome.

[a] FDA-approved.
[b] CE-approved.
[c] CLIA-waived.
[d] In development.

Box 1
Strategic planning for POCT in disaster settings: gap analysis

Discovery

Novel new POC technologies for complex POCT in different global settings

Operational characteristics

Native sample testing from complex matrices with minimal prenalytical processing

Cassette-contained sample processing to avoid (pathogen) contamination

Back-end biohazard disposal in the same cassette, which can be disposed of intact

Internal, automated, and electronic quality control; external proficiency testing

Battery operation with flexible multiple power supplies

Format, licensing, and standardization

Durable handheld and portable formats for different emergency settings

Simple, fast, smart, and easy use codified to achieve CLIA-waived status

Competency demonstrated beforehand as part of preparedness in disaster plan

Standardized test results verified with "new math" (eg, LS MAD curves)

Environmental robustness

Sensors on board to document location and environmental conditions

Durable reagents and equipment not susceptible to environmental stresses

Environmental certification based on dynamic stress testing

Suitability for meteorologic profiles of disaster sites worldwide

Diagnostic performance

Quantitative POC tests capable of satisfactory accuracy, sensitivity, and specificity

Multiplex or multiple patient testing with needs-based test clusters

Index case (eg, H1N1) and risk (eg, HIV 1/2 in emergency blood donors) identification

Broad-spectrum pathogen surveillance for hazards (eg, World Trade Center [WTC] cough)

Mutations and detection of multiresistant strains (eg, tuberculosis) in challenging environments

Knowledge optimization

Full user awareness of performance characteristics based on field evaluations

Informatics compatibility, connectivity, and archival in small-world networks

Risk indexing of diagnostic targets, wireless results reporting, and outcomes monitoring

Cost-effectiveness for implementation in low-resource settings

---

instrument was not the source of the errors. Laboratory personnel noted that when false-positive potassium critical values were seen, a hemoglobin A1C test was also ordered.

On investigation of the sample processing, Dighe and colleagues[41] found that both tubes were being packaged with ice and transported to the testing facility. Icing blood tubes has been shown to lyse red blood cells and falsely elevate potassium levels.[41] Laboratory technologists subsequently altered the transport requirement for hemoglobin A1C and observed a substantial decrease in potassium false-positive values in ensuing months.[41] When POCT devices are reliable, these types of preanalytical problems can be minimized or eliminated. To ensure best patient care, preanalytical processing methods used on field-worthy POCT devices should be self-contained and disposable, but free from confounding preanalytical errors.

Box 1 lists several other gaps that need to be addressed. For example, the introduction of locally smooth median absolute difference (LS MAD) curves as a mathematical statistical method to visually analyze the accuracy of POCT blood glucose meters shows that performance in hypoglycemic and hyperglycemic ranges of most blood glucose meters in current use exceeds error tolerance limits for adult critically ill patient populations.[42,43] POCT technologies intended for emergency and disaster settings and critically ill patient populations can be improved, standardized, and verified with this new math (see **Box 1**) to enable better performance and patient outcomes.

The search and discovery of novel new POC technologies should be actively pursued by researchers. Devices are needed in various global environments across the world. In these different conditions, POCT will encounter new challenges to be overcome. As noted above, POCT instruments must be environmentally robust and capable of withstanding dynamic stresses (see **Box 1**). In addition, POCT devices should be capable of diagnosing multiple pathogens with adequate clinical sensitivity and specificity (see **Box 1**), ideally including extensively drug-resistant tuberculosis, malaria, and influenza. New and novel POCT devices will be created in the future featuring improved operational characteristics, environmental robustness, diagnostic performance, and knowledge optimization that enable disaster responders to rapidly diagnose and treat victims and fill current technology gaps.

INTEGRATION STRATEGY: POCT AND SMALL-WORLD NETWORKS

Strategic placement of POCT devices within small-world networks (SWN) will effectively facilitate rapid evidence-based medical decisions.[5] SWNs enable information to be transmitted quickly from site to site and facilitate quick triage of patients to appropriate points of evaluation.[5] SWNs can help manage POCT operations to improve overall efficiency and cost-effectiveness by integrating health care delivery components, including home monitoring, primary care unit testing, mobile medical unit, alternate medical care site, triage, emergency room, and local hospital resources.[5]

Thus, when a disaster situation arises, such as Hurricane Katrina, the tsunami in Southeast Asia, or the novel H1N1 (swine flu) pandemic, SWNs can effectively allocate POCT resources to allow for rapid and cost-effective patient care or isolation of index cases, as needed, that is also efficient within the context of regional resources. This strategic integration of POCT into regional aspects of disaster and emergency response will ensure that patient care will be rapid and effective.

SUMMARY

Use of POCT in disaster and emergency situations will efficiently facilitate rapid evidence-based diagnosis at the site of patient care. A variety of tests are currently available for POCT in hospitals, but the spectrum of POC tests for emergency and disaster care must be broadened.

The development of pathogen test clusters, based on needs assessment survey results, must be incorporated into new POCT device designs. Besides developing innovative POCT devices, current gaps in POCT technology and availability must be filled to ensure optimal patient care wherever the patient might be.

Integration and global use of POCT in emergencies will help prevent newdemics from accelerating as seen during Hurricane Katrina and the current influenza pandemic (novel H1N1), while simultaneously improving immediate patient care.

When a disaster or emergency strikes and as POCT use becomes standard for SWN preparedness, emergency medical responders, alternate medical facilities, and hospitals will be ready to deal effectively with the crises and avoid the pitfalls of the past, when adequate POCT was not available or not used efficiently.

However, given current state-of-the-art POCT, the United States and other countries are not prepared. Having environmentally robust and rapid POCT devices that are deployable to disaster and emergency sites, and also validated for the care of the critically ill, will bring care to the point of need where physicians and nurses can make fast, evidence-based decisions for triage and treatment.

ACKNOWLEDGMENTS

The authors thank the needs assessment survey respondents for their valuable contributions. Figures and tables were provided with permission and courtesy of Knowledge Optimization, Davis, CA.

REFERENCES

1. Kost GJ, Tran NK, Tuntideelert M, et al. Katrina, the tsunami and point-of-care testing: optimizing rapid response diagnosis in disasters. Am J Clin Pathol 2006;126:513–20.
2. Diiulio R. A New Orleans hospital weathers the storm. MLO Med Lab Obs 2007; 39:18–20.
3. Katrina's death: who's to blame? The Economist 2007;13:35.
4. Kost GJ, Minear M, Siegel PM, et al. Knowledge, education, mind connectivity: using telemedicine to achieve a global vision for point-of-care testing. Point Care 2008;7:69–71.
5. Kost GJ. Newdemics, public health, small-world networks, and point-of-care testing. Point Care 2006;5:138–44.
6. Louie RF, Sumner SL, Belcher S, et al. Thermal stress and point-of-care testing performance: suitability of glucose test strips and blood gas cartridges for disaster response. Disaster Med Public Health Prep 2009;3:13–7.
7. Shaman J, Day JF, Stieglitz M. Drought-induced amplification of Saint Louis encephalitis virus, Florida. Emerg Infect Dis 2002;8:575–80.
8. Shaman J, Day JK, Stieglitz M. Drought-induced amplification and epidemic transmission of West Nile virus in southern Florida. J Med Entomol 2005;42: 134–41.
9. Bangs MJ, Subianto DB. El Nino and associated outbreaks of severe malaria in highland populations in Irian Jaya, Indonesia: a review and epidemiological perspective. Southeast Asian J Trop Med Public Health 1999;30:608–19.
10. Schneider E, Hajjeh RA, Spiegel RA, et al. A coccidioidomycosis outbreak following the Northridge, Calif, Earthquake. JAMA 1997;277:904–8.
11. Tao C, Kang M, Chen Z, et al. Microbiologic study of the pathogens isolated from wound culture among Wengchuan earthquake survivors. Diagn Microbiol Infect Dis 2009;63:268–70.
12. Bulut M, Fedakar R, Akkose S, et al. Medical experience of university hospital in Turkey after the 1999 Marmara earthquake. Emerg Med J 2005;22:494–8.
13. Kazancioglu R, Cagatay A, Colangu S, et al. The characteristics of infections in crush syndrome. Clin Microbiol Infect 2002;8:202–6.

14. Qadri F, Khan A, Faruque A, et al. Enterotoxigenic *Escherichia coli* and *Vibrio cholerae* diarrhea, Bangladesh, 2004. Emerg Infect Dis 2005;11:1104–7.

15. World Health Organization. Flooding and communicable diseases fact sheet: risk assessment and preventative measures. Available at: http://www.who.int/hac/techguidance/ems/flood_cds/en/print.html. Accessed June 24, 2009.

16. Vollaard A, Ali S, Asten H, et al. Risk factors for typhoid and paratyphoid fever in Jakarta, Indonesia. JAMA 2004;209:2607–15.

17. Vernon D, Banner W, Cantwell P, et al. *Streptococcus pneumoniae* bacteremia associated with near-drowning. Crit Care Med 1990;18:1175–6.

18. Ender P, Dolan M. Pneumonia associated with near-drowning. Clin Infect Dis 1997;25:896–907.

19. Center for Disease Control and Prevention. Update on CDC's response to Hurricane Katrina – September 19th, 2005. Available at: http://www.cdc.gov/od/Katrina/09-19-05.htm. Accessed June 24, 2009.

20. Centers for Disease Control and Prevention (CDC). *Vibrio* illnesses after Hurricane Katrina – multiple states, August – September 2005. Morb Mortal Wkly Rep 2005;54:928–31.

21. Centers for Disease Control and Prevention (CDC). Infectious disease and dermatologic conditions in evacuees and rescue workers after Hurricane Katrina—multiple states, August-September, 2005. Morb Mortal Wkly Rep 2005;54: 961–4.

22. MMWR. Norovirus outbreak among evacuees from Hurricane Katrina – Houston, TX, September 2005. Morb Mortal Wkly Rep 2005;54:1016–8.

23. Sinigalliano C, Gidley M, Shibata T, et al. Impacts of Hurricanes Katrina and Rita on the microbial landscape of the New Orleans area. Proc Natl Acad Sci U S A 2007;104:9029–34.

24. Millie M, Senkowski C, Stuart L, et al. Tornado disaster in rural Georgia: triage response, injury patterns, lessons learned. Am Surg 2000;66:223–8.

25. Lupisan S, Herva E, Sombrero L, et al. Invasive bacterial infections of children in a rural province in the central Philippines. Am J Trop Med Hyg 2000;62:341–6.

26. Hiransuthikul N, Tantisiriwat W, Lertutsahakul K, et al. Skin and soft tissue infections among tsunami survivors in Southern Thailand. Clin Infect Dis 2005;41: e93–6.

27. Uckay I, Sax H, Harbarth S, et al. Multi-resistant infections in repatriated patients after natural disasters: lessons learned from the 2004 tsunami for hospital infection control. J Hosp Infect 2008;68:1–8.

28. Rajendran P, Murugan S, Raju S, et al. Bacteriological analysis of water samples from tsunami hit coastal areas of Kanyakumari district, Tamil Nadu. Indian J Med Microbiol 2006;24:114–6.

29. Ivers LC, Ryan ET. Infectious diseases of severe weather-related and flood-related natural disasters. Curr Opin Infect Dis 2006;19:408–14.

30. Thomas PA, Brackbill R, Thalji L, et al. Respiratory and other health effects reported in children exposed to the World Trade Center disaster of 11 September 2001. Environ Health Perspect 2008;116:1383–90.

31. de la Hoz RE, Christie J, Teamer JA, et al. Reflux symptoms and disorders and pulmonary disease in former World Trade Center rescue and recovery workers and volunteers. J Occup Environ Med 2008;50:1351–4.

32. Farfel M, DiGrande L, Brackbill R, et al. An overview of 9/11 experiences and respiratory and mental health conditions among World Trade Center health registry enrollees. J Urban Health 2008;85:880–909.

33. Lam C, Waldhorn R, Toner E, et al. The prospect of using alternative medical care facilities in an influenza pandemic. Biosecur Bioterror 2006;4:384–90.
34. Ginocchio CC, Lotlikar M, Falk L, et al. Clinical performance of the 3M Rapid Detection Flu A+B Test compared to R-mix culture, DFA, and BinaxNow Influenza A+B Test. J Clin Virol 2009;45:146–9.
35. Grondhal B, Puppe W, Weigl J, et al. Comparison of the BD Directigin Flu A+B kit and the Abbott TestPack RSV with a multiplex RT-PCR ELISA for rapid detection of influenza viruses and respiratory synctial virus. Clin Microbiol Infect 2005;11: 848–50.
36. Hurt AC, Alexander R, Hibbert J, et al. Performance of six influenza rapid tests in detecting human influenza in clinical specimens. J Clin Virol 2007;39:132–5.
37. Cazacu AC, Demmler GJ, Neuman MA, et al. Comparison of a new lateral-flow chromatographic membrane immunoassay to viral culture for rapid detection and differentiation of influenza A and B viruses in respiratory specimens. J Clin Microbiol 2004;42:3661–4.
38. Pabbaraju K, Tokaryk KL, Wong S, et al. Comparison of the Luminex xTAG respiratory viral panel with in-house nucleic acid amplification tests for diagnosis of respiratory virus infections. J Clin Microbiol 2008;46:3056–62.
39. Nishiura H, Wilson N, Baker MG. Quarantine for pandemic influenza control at the borders of small island nations. BMC Infect Dis 2009;9:27 [Published online March 11, 2009]. Doi:10.1186/1471-2334-9-27.
40. Grandjean L, Moore DA. Tuberculosis in the developing world: recent advances in diagnosis with special consideration of extensively drug-resistant tuberculosis. Curr Opin Infect Dis 2008;21:454–61.
41. Dighe AS, Jones JB, Parham S, et al. Survey of critical value reporting and reduction of false-positive critical value results. Arch Pathol Lab Med 2008;132: 1666–71.
42. Kost GJ, Tran NK, Sifontes JR, et al. Locally smoothed median absolute difference curves and the first global performance cooperative. Point Care 2009;8: 45–52.
43. Kost GJ, Tran NK, Louie RF, et al. Assessing the performance of handheld glucose testing for critical care. Diabetes Technol Ther 2008;10:445–51.

Selected Topics in Point-of-Care Testing: Whole Blood Creatinine, Influenza Testing, Fetal Fibronectin and Patient Self-testing in the Home

Kent Lewandrowski, MD

KEYWORDS

- Point-of-care • Influenza • Creatinine • Fetal
- Fibronectin • Home testing

POINT-OF-CARE ASSAYS FOR CREATININE

Measurement of creatinine is the most common method employed to assess renal function and to measure or estimate the glomerular filtration rate. In the past, most laboratories reported the serum, plasma and/or urine creatinine value as a simple number, requiring clinicians to use formulas or nomograms to determine the creatinine clearance if desired. The problem with this approach was that clinicians often did not perform these calculations. However, it is well known that use of the creatinine value alone is a less than optimal approach to assess renal function and this inadequacy is greater in patients with renal dysfunction.[1]

Many factors influence the measured creatinine value and the normal range varies depending on gender, age, body weight and other variables. In recent years, a number of laboratories have begun reporting creatinine values along with an estimated creatinine clearance (eGFR) based on a formula originally validated by the Modification of Diet in Renal Disease Study.[1] This formula uses information normally readily available in the laboratory computer information system, including the patients age and gender. The results are usually reported with a correction factor to account for racial

Massachusetts General Hospital, Harvard Medical School, 55 Fruit Street, Gray 5 Chemistry, Boston, MA 02114, USA
E-mail address: klewandrowski@partners.org

Clin Lab Med 29 (2009) 607–614
doi:10.1016/j.cll.2009.07.013
0272-2712/09/$ – see front matter © 2009 Elsevier Inc. All rights reserved.

differences. The typical reference range reported for the eGFR is greater than 60 mL/min/1.73m.[2]

Recently, several companies have developed point-of-care creatinine assays—either as stand-alone tests or as part of routine chemistry panels such as the basic metabolic panel. These assays are based on the same analytical methods that are used on traditional chemistry analyzers. Some devices are also equipped with software to calculate the eGFR. Development of these new point-of-care assays using whole blood or plasma has permitted consideration of when it might be desirable to perform rapid creatinine testing at the bedside. Scenarios in which point-of care testing (POCT) might have an advantage include:

1. Nephrology clinics following patients with renal disease.
2. Settings where rapid measurement of routine chemistry tests, such as the basic metabolic panel, are deemed desirable including emergency departments and critical care units.
3. Radiology departments where patients may be administered contrast agents. Patients with renal dysfunction are at increased risk for both contrast-induced acute kidney injury and for nephrogenic systemic sclerosis. In busy radiology centers, the ability to determine a rapid creatinine value and eGFR avoids costly delays while waiting for centralized laboratory test results.

The relative merits of POCT for each of these applications are discussed below.

Nephrology Clinics: Most patients being followed in nephrology clinics will require regular determination of creatinine levels. However, virtually all of these patients will receive other laboratory tests that are also necessary for their overall evaluation. For this reason, the benefit of providing only a creatinine value in the absence of other tests is of dubious value unless the creatinine is performed along with other key tests to permit immediate adjustments to treatment during the same office visit.

Applications of the Basic Metabolic Panel: The basic metabolic panel is one of the most common tests performed in emergency departments and acute care settings. Logically, a rapid point-of-care panel would have significant value. Prior to the development of POC creatinine tests, a number of companies offered products capable of performing electrolytes along with arterial blood gases. Several studies evaluated the clinical and operational benefits of these devices in the emergency setting.[2,3] For example, Parvin and colleagues[2] evaluated five analytes (sodium, potassium, chloride, glucose and urea nitrogen) and found no impact on emergency department length of stay (ED LOS). Kendall and colleagues[3] studied the benefits of emergency department testing using point-of-care testing for electrolytes, hematocrit and blood gases. They reported that in some cases medical decisions were made more rapidly, but they could not demonstrate an impact on ED LOS. Part of the reason for this apparent failure of POCT to have a positive impact on ED operations is that the menu of tests offered was not complete. Other tests were sent to the central laboratory to complete the evaluation of the patient.

The basic metabolic panel is one of the most common tests ordered in the emergency department[4] and, indeed, in a number of acute care settings. The tests included in the panel are sodium, potassium, chloride, total CO_2, glucose, creatinine and calcium. Offering a complete panel in a POCT format creates an opportunity for caregivers to obtain rapid whole blood results for these commonly ordered tests. The development of whole blood creatinine assays completed the menu for this panel. Whether this development translates into a new opportunity for POCT remains to be seen. The basic metabolic panel is often co-ordered with a complete blood count, liver function panel, coagulation studies and other tests.[4] The essential feature for a point-of-care technology to impact clinical operations is that the testing either:

1. Impacts a key decision point during a clinical event (eg, cardiac markers, D-dimer);
2. Or the testing offers a complete menu for the clinical situation in question such that all required testing is performed directly at the bedside without waiting for other test results to return from the central laboratory.

It is not yet clear that the basic metabolic panel performed at the point-of-care, in the absence of other testing such as the complete blood count, will have sufficient leverage to have a beneficial impact on clinical operations.

Applications in Radiology: Perhaps the single most important application for point-of-care testing for creatinine lies in the radiology department where patients are administered contrast agents prior to computed tomographic (CT) or magnetic resonance imaging (MRI) scans. Administration of intravenous iodinated CT contrast media is a common cause of acute kidney injury (contrast induced nephropathy [CIN]).[5] The acute kidney injury presumably results from renal ischemia and from direct toxic effects to the renal tubular epithelium.[5] Most intravenous contrast agents have been reported to cause CIN, including those used for applications other than CT, such as cardiac catheterization. Contrast induced nephropathy has been defined as either a >25% increase in the serum creatinine or an increase in creatinine of 0.5 mg/dL following administration of the agent.[6] Most cases of contrast induced nephropathy occur within 24–48 hours.[5] Major risk factors include preexisting renal dysfunction as manifested by an eGFR < 60 mL/min/1.73m,[2] patients with diabetes mellitus, and reduced effective circulating volume. Various approaches have been described to prevent CIN as reviewed by Sterling and colleagues.[5]

Patient flow in busy radiology departments is dependent on a number of factors. In patients who are about to receive intravenous contrast agents, it is important to know the status of their renal function prior to the procedure. In many cases, this information is not known by the radiology staff at the time the patient presents to the radiology service. Drawing a specimen to be sent to the clinical laboratory for serum/plasma creatinine introduces significant delay and impairs the efficient operation of the service. The availability of rapid whole blood point-of-care creatinine testing with calculation of the eGFR eliminates this problem and allows consideration of preventive measures for patients identified with chronic renal dysfunction.

Nephrogenic systemic fibrosis is a rare complication occurring after the administration of gadolinium-containing MRI contrast agents.[7] This complication appears to occur only in patients with moderate to severe kidney dysfunction. The risk of nephrogenic systemic fibrosis is minimal in patients with an eGFR > 30 mL/min/1.73m.[2] In patients with an unknown renal function status, point-of-care testing for creatinine with calculation of the eGFR is a practical alternative to sending specimens to a central laboratory with the resultant delays in commencing the procedure.

POINT-OF-CARE ASSAYS FOR INFLUENZA A AND B

Influenza A and B are respiratory viruses that cause seasonal outbreaks, usually in the fall or winter seasons in temperate zones or year-round in tropical climates. Influenza A, but not B, is also responsible for occasional worldwide pandemics. Typically influenza A produces more servere outbreaks. The designation of influenza A versus B is based on the antigenic characteristics of the nucleoprotein (NP) and matrix protein (M). Influenza A is further subtyped based on its surface hemagglutinin antigen (H) and neuraminidase antigen (N). The hemagglutinin is the site for viral binding to the cell surface whereas the neuraminidase degrades the receptor and plays a role in viral release from infected cells. Only H1, H2, H3, N1 and N2 are associated with major epidemics. Following infection, humans develop antibodies to both the H and N antigens. Antibodies to the H antigen are a significant factor in developing immunity whereas antibodies to the N antigen reduce infection and spread of the virus.

The H and N antigens of influenza exhibit periodic changes in their antigenic composition. Minor changes have been designated as "antigenic drift" and may occur with both influenza A and B. Conversely, major changes in antigenicity have been termed "antigenic shifts" and only occur with influenza A. Antigenic shifts presumably result from gene reassortments between human and animal influenza viruses and may cause major pandemics.

Interpersonal transmission of influenza virus occurs by spread of respiratory droplets expelled from infected patients by coughing and sneezing. Transmission may also occur by hand contact with infected surfaces followed by touching of the nose and mouth. Treatment of influenza with appropriate antiviral agents has been shown to reduce the duration of symptoms only if the drugs are administered early in the course of symptomatic infection. For this reason, rapid diagnosis of infected patients is essential to making appropriate decisions concerning antiviral treatment. It is also important to differentiate influenza A and B, both for epidemiologic reasons and because the treatment of the two viruses may be different.

Various laboratory methods are available for the diagnosis of influenza as shown in **Table 1**. Some of these methods, such as viral culture and polymerase chain reaction (PCR), take too much time to obtain a result to be clinically practical. Others such as direct fluorescent antibody testing (DFA) can achieve results compatible with the timing of clinical decision-making, but this method requires skilled technologists to perform testing. Furthermore, DFA testing is impractical to perform on a 24-hour, 7-day per week basis.

Table 1
Abbreviated Centers For Disease Control (CDC) listing of laboratory testing for influenza

Test	Influenza Types Detected	Specimens	Time to Result	Rapid Test Available
Viral culture	A and B	NP swab, throat swab, nasal wash, bronchial wash, nasal aspirate, sputum	5–10 days	No
DFA	A and B	NP swab, nasal wash, bronchial wash, nasal aspirate, sputum	2–4 hours	No
RT-PCR	A and B	NP swab, throat swab, nasal wash, bronchial wash, nasal aspirate, sputum	1–2 days	No
EIA	A and B	NP swab, throat swab, nasal wash, bronchial wash	2 hours	No
Rapid tests	A and B	NP swab and other	<30 minutes	Yes

Finally, most patients who have influenza present to outpatient locations that do not have on-site laboratory support. For these reasons, rapid POCT has significant appeal.

A different situation occurs in hospital emergency departments where patients may present with severe acute influenza. Some of these patients, particularly the elderly, have other medical conditions and will be admitted to the hospital. Admitting patients with influenza (or other transmissible respiratory viruses) raises issues of infection control as shown in **Table 2**. Depending on the virus, droplet and/or contact precautions may be necessary. A major issue occurs when hospitals are full to capacity and inpatient beds are scarce. In this situation, it is important to know if the patient has a respiratory virus and, if so, which one. Knowing the cause of the illness allows proper precautions to be instituted and, in some cases, patients with the same virus can be cohorted in the same room. The typical respiratory virus panel in microbiology laboratories includes influenza A and B, parainfluenza virus, respiratory syncytial virus, adenovirus, and metapneumovirus. In microbiology laboratories in major hospitals, the testing is usually performed using a direct immunofluoresence test that can detect all six viruses. However, this test requires several hours to perform and is rarely available on evening and night shifts. The potentially long wait for test results complicates the management of patients awaiting admission in a busy emergency department. In this setting, the availability of rapid POCT is potentially useful.

A number of point-of-care tests for viral pathogens are available, including tests for influenza A and B, RSV and adenovirus. When performed by trained personnel on properly collected specimens, many of these tests are highly specific (99%), albeit their sensitivity varies and is often in the range of 67%–82%.[8,9] For this reason, a positive test is usually reliable, but negative test results cannot be used to exclude influenza infection. A second important caveat is that point-of-care tests are not configured to evaluate for a panel of respiratory viruses. Therefore, a negative test result for influenza A and B does not exclude other potentially important respiratory viruses. When these rapid tests are used in an emergency department setting to evaluate patients who are going to be admitted to an inpatient bed, a positive result is very informative, but a negative test provides little actionable information.

FETAL FIBRONECTIN

Fetal fibronectin (FFN) is an immunologically distinct member of the fibronectin family of proteins that may play a role in attachment of the fetal trophoblast to the maternal decidual surface. An excellent review of FFN and its use in clinical practice is provided by Grenache and Gronowski.[10] FFN can be measured by immunoassay. The assay currently approved by the US Food and Drug Administration employs a single use disposable cartridge and a small benchtop analyzer. The test may be performed in the central laboratory or at the point-of-care in the obstetrics unit or physicians office. FFN has been shown to be useful in the following settings:[10]

1. Prediction of preterm delivery with a high negative predictive value. The positive predictive value of the test is less reliable;

Table 2				
Isolation procedures for respiratory viruses at the Massachusetts general hospital				
	Influenza	Parainfluenza	Adenovirus	RSV
Contact	No	Yes	Yes	Yes
Droplet	Yes	No	Yes	No

2. As an aid to guide management of preterm labor. A negative FFN test suggests that tocolytic therapy can be avoided;
3. Prediction of term labor. A positive FFN test indicates probable delivery within 48 hours;
4. Prediction of preterm delivery in twin gestation in symptomatic (not asymptomatic) patients.

All of the settings listed above have proven clinically challenging, based on patient history and physical examination. As a result, when rapid testing for FFN became commercially available, the test quickly became standard of care in hospitals in the United States. In many respects, FFN testing is an excellent example of how a point-of-care test targeted to a specific clinical problem can improve patient management and outcomes.

PATIENT SELF-TESTING IN THE HOME

Patient self-testing in the home setting is well established for diabetic patients to mange their glucose values and adjust insulin therapy. In the past, this testing involved older technologies, such as urine dipstick tests for glucose or semi-quantitative measurements of blood glucose. The development of small hand held glucose meters that used a capillary fingerstick blood sample to produce a quantitative glucose value revolutionized the management of diabetes mellitus. These devices made it possible for patients to achieve tight glycemic control on an ongoing basis and this has been linked to improved long- term outcomes for diabetic patients. For example, the Diabetes Control and Complications Trial Research Group demonstrated that intensive therapy delayed the onset and slowed the progression of diabetic retinopathy, nephropathy and neuropathy in patients with type 1 diabetes (formerly insulin dependant diabetes mellitus, [IDDM]).[11] The UKPDS 33 trial of intensive therapy in type 2 diabetes demonstrated a significant reduction in microvascular complications of diabetes.[12] As a result of these and other studies, the benefits of intensive therapy made possible by home quantitative blood glucose testing have become clear.[13]

Another area of testing where self-testing at home has been shown to improve therapy is in the management of anticoagulation. In a study by Sawicki using an anti-coagulation education program that included self-management demonstrated that home testing was associated with improved accuracy of anticoagulation control when compared to conventional management in the physicians office.[14]

A number of other laboratory tests are sold over-the-counter in the United States as shown in **Box 1**. The trend towards making more tests available in the home setting reflects a greater appreciation of consumerism in this country and parallels the movement of more drugs (eg, nonsteroidal anti-inflammatory drugs, proton pump inhibitors) and devices (thermometers, blood pressure cuffs) towards over-the-counter sales. In all likelihood, this trend will continue.

The potential appeal to consumers of over the counter point-of-care tests is easy to appreciate. For example, if a person thought they might be pregnant there would be two possible choices:

1. Call their primary care provider for an appointment, wait several days, then take time off from work to go to the physician, be subjected to a gynecological examination, and finally get a pregnancy test. The patient might even have to tender an insurance co-pay for the visit or pay all of the cost out-of-pocket;
2. Go to the local pharmacy and purchase an inexpensive urine pregnancy test.

| Box 1 |
| Examples of over the counter home self use point-of-care tests |

1. Blood glucose testing

2. Prothrombin time/INR

3. Urine pregnancy testing

4. Fecal occult blood

5. Cholesterol

6. Drugs of abuse testing

7. Alcohol testing

8. Urinary tract infection screen

9. Infertility testing (LH)

Abbreviation: LH, lentinizing hormone

From the perspective of laboratory professionals, self-testing by patients raises a number of concerns. First is the analytical quality of the test result. The fact that a test is readily available does not necessarily mean that the device performs at an acceptable level for medical decision-making. For example, devices are sold over the counter to screen for urinary tract infection (UTI) using a urine nitrate dipstick test. Taken alone, in the absence of other laboratory data, the nitrate test itself is not able to exclude infection by a number of organisms.[15] A patient with a negative test result might erroneously conclude that they were free of infection, delay treatment, and possibly develop a more advanced UTI such as pyelonephritis. A second issue concerns training materials supplied with over-the-counter tests, which are used to teach patients the correct method of performing the testing and how to interprete the results. In the most extreme example, a patient who is not literate could purchase testing supplies and perform the test without any training having occurred. Third, the testing supplies could potentially be purchased and be stored inappropriately rendering the test result invalid. Finally, in the case of some tests, such as drugs of abuse testing, there exists significant potential for mischievous usage of the test such as illicit testing of family members or the use of drugs of abuse tests to self-screen individuals prior to employer drug screening or routine screening in rehabilitation programs. For all of these reasons, regulators need to carefully consider the benefits versus the potential downside of permitting point-of-care tests to be sold directly to consumers over the counter without a prescription.

REFERENCES

1. Levey AS, Bosch JP, Lewis JB, et al. A more accurate method to estimate glomerular filtration rate from serum creatinine: a new prediction equation. Modification of Diet in Renal Disease Study Group. Ann Intern Med 1999;130:461–70.
2. Parvin C, Lo S, Deuser S, et al. Impact of point-of-care testing on patient's length of stay in a large emergency department. Clin Chem 1996;42:711–7.
3. Kendall J, Reeves B, Clancy M. Point-of-care testing: randomized controlled trial of clinical outcome. Br Med J 1998;316:1052–7.
4. Johnson M, Lewandrowski K. Analysis of emergency department test ordering patterns in an urban academic medical center: can the point-of-care option in

a satellite laboratory provide sufficient menu to permit full service testing. Point of Care 2007;6:134–8.

5. Sterling K, Tehrani T, Rudnick M. Clinical significance and preventive strategies for contrast induced nephropathy. Curr Opin Nephrol Hypertens 2008;17:616–23.

6. Barrett B, Parfrey P. Clinical practice. Preventing nephropathy induced by contrast medium. N Engl J Med 2006;354:379–86.

7. Prince M, Zhang H, Morris M, et al. Incidence of nephrogenic systemic fibrosis at two large medical centers. Radiology 2008;248:807–16.

8. Poehling K, Zhu Y, Tang Y, et al. Accuracy and impact of a point-of-care rapid influenza test in young children with respiratory illnessess. Arch Pediatr Adolesc Med 2006;160:713–8.

9. Weitzel T, Schnabel E, Dieckmann S, et al. Evaluation of a new point-of-care test for influenza A and B in travellors with influenza-like symptoms. Clin Microbiol Infect 2007;13:665–9.

10. Grenache D, Gronowski A. Fetal fibronectin (chapter18). In: Nichols J, editor. Point-of-care testing. Performance improvement and evidence based outcomes. New York: Marcel Dekker; 2003. p. 477–89.

11. DCCT Research Group. The effect of intensive treatment of diabetes on the development and progression of long-term complications in insulin-dependent diabetes mellitus. N Engl J Med 1993;329:977–86.

12. UKPDS 33 Research Group. Intensive blood-glucose control with sulphonylureas or insulin compared with conventional treatment and risk of complications in patients with type 2 diabetes. Lancet 1998;352:837–53.

13. Price C. Regular review: point of care testing. BMJ 2001;322:1285–8.

14. Sawicki P. A structured teaching and self management program for patients receiving oral anticoagulation: a randomized controlled trial. JAMA 1999;281: 145–50.

15. Holloway J, Joshi N, O'bryan T. Positive urine nitrate test: an accurate predictor of absence of pure enterococcal bacteria. Southern Med J 2000;93:681–2.

Index

Note: Page numbers of article titles are in **boldface** type.

A

Accumetrics device, for platelet function testing, 544–546
Activated clotting time, 548–549
Acute coronary syndromes, cardiac marker testing for, 561–568
Adenovirus testing, 611
Aggregation, platelet, 543
Amniotic fluid, microscopic detection of, 575
Anticoagulation therapy, monitoring of. *See* Coagulation testing.
Aspirin resistance, 544–546
Automation, of molecular diagnostic tests, 555–560

B

Basic metabolic panel, 608–609
Billing, 446–447
Blood, occult. *See* Fecal occult blood testing.
B-natriuretic peptide testing, for congestive heart failure, 568–569

C

Cancer, colorectal, screening for. *See* Fecal occult blood testing.
Cardiac marker testing, **561–571**
　　for acute coronary syndromes, 561–568
　　for congestive heart failure, 568–569
　　in emergency department, 485
Casts, urine, 579
Cellulose tape method, for pinworm collection, 577–578
Centralization, of POCT, 436–439
Chest pain, cardiac marker testing for, 561–568
Chromosomal instability, in cancer, fecal DNA testing for, 530, 533–536
Clearview HIV tests, 492–494
Clinical Laboratory Improvement Amendments (CLIA) of 1988 certificates
　　categories of, 464–465
　　CMS-deemed status of, 468–472, 474–475
　　control procedures for, 467, 473
　　inspections for, 474
　　moderate-complexity testing under, 466, 470–472
　　personnel involved in, 466, 469, 471
　　procedure manuals for, 467, 469–470
　　proficiency testing for, 469, 471, 473
　　quality systems for, 473–474

Clin Lab Med 29 (2009) 615–622
doi:10.1016/S0272-2712(09)00096-1
0272-2712/09/$ – see front matter © 2009 Elsevier Inc. All rights reserved.

Moving?

Make sure your subscription moves with you!

To notify us of your new address, find your **Clinics Account Number** (located on your mailing label above your name), and contact customer service at:

Email: journalscustomerservice-usa@elsevier.com

800-654-2452 (subscribers in the U.S. & Canada)
314-447-8871 (subscribers outside of the U.S. & Canada)

Fax number: 314-447-8029

Elsevier Health Sciences Division
Subscription Customer Service
3251 Riverport Lane
Maryland Heights, MO 63043

*To ensure uninterrupted delivery of your subscription, please notify us at least 4 weeks in advance of move.

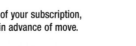